MOTHERS, BABIES, AND DISEASE IN LATER LIFE

MOTHERS, BABIES, AND DISEASE IN LATER LIFE

D J P Barker, BSc, PhD, MD, FRCP, FRCOG, FFPHM
Director, MRC Environmental Epidemiology Unit,
Professor of Clinical Epidemiology, University of Southampton,
Consultant Physician, Royal South Hants Hospital

BMJ
Publishing
Group

First published in 1994
by the BMJ Publishing Group, BMA House, Tavistock Square,
London WC1H 9JR

British Library Cataloguing in Publication Data

A catalogue record for this book is available
from the British Library

ISBN 0-7279-0835-9

Typeset, printed, and bound in Great Britain by
Latimer Trend & Company Ltd, Plymouth

Contents

Preface

This book describes how the nourishment a baby receives from its mother, and its exposure to infection after birth, determine its susceptibility to disease in later life. Its theme is that improving the nutrition and health of girls and young women, and of mothers during pregnancy and lactation, will improve the health of their children throughout their lives.

Geographical studies first suggested that if a baby is undernourished it becomes susceptible to coronary heart disease and stroke in adult life, and chapter 1 reviews them. Chapter 2, written with Yasmin Sultan, attempts a comprehensive review of animal studies which have shown that under-nutrition in early life permanently "programs" the body's structure and metabolism. Chapters 3 to 6 describe studies in humans which show that impaired growth in the womb and during infancy is followed by coronary heart disease, diabetes, hypertension, raised serum cholesterol, and abnormal blood clotting in later life. Chapter 7 describes how poor lung growth before birth, and respiratory infection during infancy, determine susceptibility to chronic bronchitis. Descriptions of acute appendicitis and Paget's disease of bone in chapter 8 illustrate how other infections in infancy and early childhood may be linked to later disease.

Chapter 9 outlines the complex processes by which a mother nourishes her baby, and chapter 10 describes how the poor health of people who are in lower socioeconomic groups, or who live in certain areas, can be linked to past neglect of the welfare of mothers and babies. Chapter 11 discusses strategies for the future, and suggests that further research into the nutrition and health of mothers and babies may lead to better prevention of disease in future generations and to better treatment of disease in generations already born.

In this book I have referred extensively to the work of my colleagues in the MRC Environmental Epidemiology Unit at the University of Southampton, and it is a pleasure to acknowledge them. Clive Osmond played a central role in developing our research programme. Adrian Bull, David Coggon, Cyrus Cooper, Caroline Fall, Martin Gardner, Keith Godfrey, Catherine Law, Barrie Margetts, Christopher Martyn, Brian Pannett, David Phillips, Sian Robinson, Seif Shaheen, and Paul Winter all made important scientific contributions. Others in the Unit have helped with the fieldwork, data analysis, and administrative support, and I am grateful to them all. Our studies were possible because of the vision of doctors and nurses who compiled detailed records on babies many years ago, and through the generosity of the men, women, and children who were those babies and who have taken part in our surveys. Without the help of the staff at the NHS Central Register in Southport it would not have been possible to trace people from birth to adult life.

It is a pleasure to acknowledge the help of others working in this field: Professor Nick Hales and Dr Alan Lucas at the University of Cambridge; Professor Tom Meade at the MRC Epidemiology and Medical Care Unit; Professor Chris Edwards and Dr Jonathan Seckl at the University of Edinburgh; Professor Peter Gluckman and Dr Jane Harding at the University of Auckland, New Zealand; Professor Jeffrey Robinson and Dr Julie Owens at the University of Adelaide, Australia; and my colleagues Professor Alan Jackson and Mr Tim Wheeler at the University of Southampton.

The MRC has taken a lead in developing research into the maternal and fetal origins of adult disease and I am grateful to the staff at MRC Head Office in London who have enabled this. Major financial support has come from the Wellcome Trust, the British Heart Foundation, the Dunhill Trust, Wellbeing, Children Nationwide, and the Wessex Medical Trust.

The development of a new field of research is greatly helped by the interest of a major journal. The *BMJ* published many of the earlier papers on programming and adult disease, and in 1992 published a collection of them under the title *Fetal and Infant Origins of Adult Disease*. The BMJ Publishing Group is now publishing this book. Acknowledging the important role of the *BMJ* and its editor, Dr Richard Smith, gives me the opportunity also to thank the many BMJ staff who make their authors' task so much easier.

This book was typed by Linda Bennett and Linda Fairley, edited by Shirley Simmonds, and assisted in innumerable ways by Hilary Brenan. It would not have been written without the help of my wife, Jan, who also made the embroidery for the book cover.

D J P BARKER
Southampton, 1994

1: Clues from geography

The three babies in fig 1.1 were born in the same hospital last year. Each was born after an uncomplicated pregnancy and delivery, and had a birthweight within the normal range. Yet the findings which will be described in this book suggest that the baby on the left, the smallest one, will be more susceptible to coronary heart disease, stroke, diabetes, and chronic bronchitis as an adult, and is destined to have a shorter, less healthy life.

The thesis of this book is that a baby's nourishment before birth, and during infancy, and its exposure to infection during early childhood, influence the diseases it will develop in later life. Chapters 3–6 examine the long term effects of early nutrition; chapters 7 and 8 examine the effects of infection; chapter 9 reviews the control of fetal growth; and chapters 10 and 11 discuss the implications of these observations for the prevention of disease.

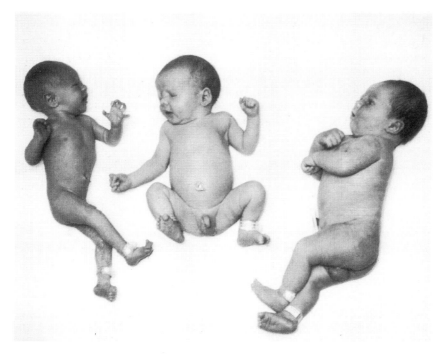

FIG 1.1—*Three newborn babies.*

Early clues to the possible importance of early life in determining adult diseases came from studies of differences in disease rates occurring between one place and another, or at different times. This chapter focuses on coronary heart disease and stroke, together known as cardiovascular disease. Later chapters describe the geographical distributions and time trends of other diseases, including diabetes, chronic bronchitis, and acute appendicitis.

At the start of this century the incidence of coronary heart disease rose steeply; it rapidly became the most common cause of death in Western countries. Its incidence is now rising in other parts of the world – India, China, and Russia. As such rapid increases in incidence over a short time cannot be the result of changes in gene frequency, attention was directed at the environment, in particular the lifestyles of men and women in industrialised countries.

Given that the other major heart disorder in adult life, chronic rheumatic heart disease, was already known to be caused by events in childhood, it may seem surprising that adults rather than children were the early focus of research into coronary heart disease. Perhaps the discovery of the powerful effects of cigarette smoking on lung cancer directed attention in this way. Whatever the reason for this focus, 40 years of research into adult lifestyle have met with limited success in explaining the origins of coronary heart disease: cigarette smoking and obesity have been implicated; evidence on dietary fat has accumulated to the point where a public health policy of reduced intake is prudent, though unproven; much, however, remains unexplained.

In many Western countries the steep rise of coronary heart disease was followed by a fall; in the USA,[1] this was of the order of one quarter in the last 20 years. No parallel changes in adult lifestyle seem to explain this. In Britain there were large changes in lifestyle during the Second World War, especially in diet, but there were no corresponding changes in incidence of coronary heart disease. Government food policy led to major and widespread changes in diet, so that fat and sugar consumption fell sharply and fibre consumption rose.[2 3] Death rates from coronary heart disease in middle aged men and women, however, continued to rise throughout the war and the period of post-war rationing.[4]

The geography of coronary heart disease in Britain is paradoxical. Rates are twice as high in the poorer areas of the country, and in lower income groups.[5] The steep rise of the disease in Britain and other Western countries was associated with rising prosperity,[6 7] so why should its rates be lowest in the most prosperous places, such as London and the home counties, and in the highest income groups?[8 9] Biochemical and physiological measurements in adult life, including serum cholesterol and blood pressure, have been shown to be linked to coronary heart disease.[10] Yet, even when combined with these risk factors, adult lifestyle has limited ability to predict

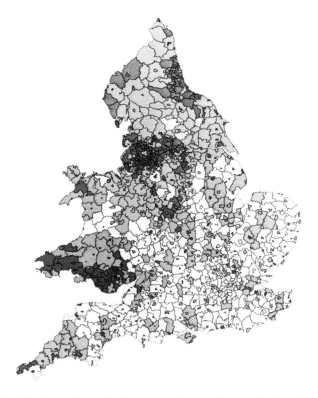

FIG 1.2—*Standardised mortality ratios for coronary heart disease in England and Wales among men aged 35–74 years during 1968–78.* ■ *high;* ▦ *medium;* □ *low.*

coronary heart disease.[11] Rose[12] has pointed out that, for a man falling into the lowest risk groups for cigarette smoking, serum cholesterol concentrations, blood pressure, and pre-existing symptoms of coronary heart disease, the most common cause of death is coronary heart disease.

It is, perhaps, surprising that geographical studies gave the early clue that answers to these paradoxes might come from events *in utero*. Nevertheless, the first indication that coronary heart disease might be linked to impaired fetal growth came from the demonstration that differences in rates of death from coronary heart disease in different parts of England and Wales paralleled past differences in death rates among newborn babies.[13] In these early studies the death certificates for all people who had died in England and Wales during 1968–78 were used to calculate coronary heart disease rates for men and women in each of the 1366 local authority areas.[14] Death rates were expressed as standardised mortality ratios which take into account differences in the age and sex distribution of populations in different areas, and are calculated so that the national average is 100.

3

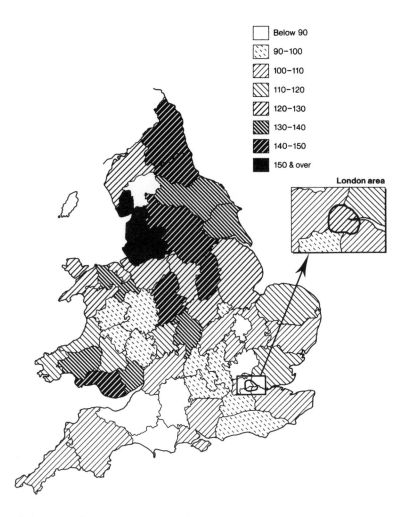

FIG 1.3—*Infant mortality rates per 1000 births in England and Wales during 1901–10.*

Fig 1.2 shows how the concentration of low mortality from coronary heart disease in the south and east contrasts with the high mortality in the northern industrial towns, and the poorer rural areas in the north and west. This contrast is seen in men and women, with the exception of north Wales where mortality among women is low.[14]

Fig 1.3 shows infant mortality (deaths under one year of age) at the turn of the century. The distribution is surprisingly similar to that of coronary heart disease today. To compare the distribution more formally, the country was divided into the 212 areas used by the Registrar General, comprising each large town (county borough), the London boroughs, the smaller towns

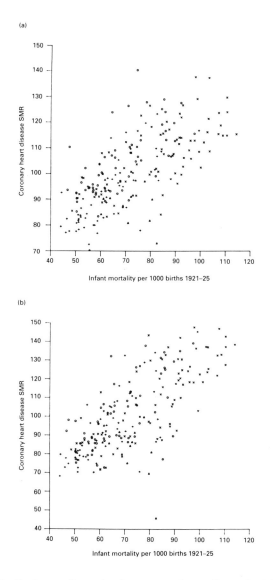

FIG 1.4—*Standardised mortality ratios for coronary heart disease in (a) men and (b) women during 1968–78 and infant mortality during 1921–25 in England and Wales.*

in each county combined together, and the rural areas in each county combined. The scattergrams in fig 1.4 confirm the similarity of the distribution of coronary heart disease and the past distribution of infant mortality. The correlation coefficient for this relationship is 0·69 in men and 0·73 in women. In separate analyses for men and women, living in large towns, small towns, or rural areas, the correlation coefficient ranged from 0·65 to 0·75.[13] Analyses based on infant mortality in an earlier period (1911 onwards) gave similar results.

Of the 23 common causes of adult death other than coronary heart disease, only chronic bronchitis, stomach cancer, and chronic rheumatic heart disease had a similarly close geographical relationship with past infant mortality. Such a relationship with infant mortality would be expected for these diseases, because they are linked to poor social conditions; their rates, like those of infant mortality, have declined during this century. The relationship between coronary heart disease and infant mortality is a paradox, however, because the rates have increased during this century.

One possible explanation of fig 1.4 is that the poor social conditions which caused infant deaths in the past are in some way linked to adult lifestyles which cause death from coronary heart disease. The nature of such a link is not, however, apparent. Differences in cigarette smoking do not appear to follow those of past infant mortality because the distribution of deaths from lung cancer is strikingly different from that of past infant mortality. Therefore it cannot be argued that the social conditions giving rise to infant death led to higher cigarette smoking in later life and hence to raised heart disease rates. Similarly, differences in dietary fat consumption do not have the same geographical distribution as past infant mortality.[15] The close geographical similarity between past infant mortality and current mortality from coronary heart disease is most easily reconciled with the opposing time trends through the hypothesis that adverse environmental influences in childhood, associated with poor living standards, directly increase susceptibility to the disease.

The environment during childhood

Findings from other studies support this general hypothesis. Forsdahl[16] reported that arteriosclerotic heart disease correlated with past infant mortality in the 20 counties of Norway, and he was the first to suggest that a poor standard of living in childhood and adolescence was a risk factor in heart disease. Another study compared east and west Finland and came to similar conclusions: that poor living conditions in childhood, with bad housing and recurrent exposure to infection, increased the later risk of coronary heart disease.[17] In the USA, in 17 states mortality from coronary heart disease was shown to be related to infant mortality resulting from diarrhoeal disease.[18]

Other observations which suggest that influences in childhood are linked to coronary heart disease include those made by Rose.[19] He reported that siblings of patients with coronary heart disease had stillbirth and infant mortality rates that were twice as high as those of controls. He concluded that "ischaemic heart disease tends to occur in individuals who come from a constitutionally weaker stock", a conclusion foreshadowing what is known today. Marmot's[20] study of London civil servants showed that death rates were higher in those who were shorter in stature, and had therefore had a worse environment in early life. Among long term employees of the Bell System Company in the USA, men whose parents had been in "white collar" occupations had a lower incidence of coronary heart disease than those from "blue collar" families.[21]

The environment *in utero*

The size of the study in England and Wales, based on almost one million deaths from coronary heart disease, together with the remarkably complete and detailed infant mortality records, made it possible to examine whether coronary heart disease is associated with specific causes of infant death and hence with particular aspects of the early environment. Infant deaths were divided into neonatal (deaths in the first month of life) and postneonatal (deaths from one month to one year). They were also divided into five causes, using a classification devised 50 years ago for an extensive analysis of the social causes of infant mortality:[22] congenital, bronchitis and pneumonia, infectious diseases, diarrhoea, and "other".

Although, using correlation coefficients, coronary heart disease has an equally strong association with either neonatal or postneonatal mortality, examination of the data suggested a closer relationship with neonatal mortality. The 15 boroughs of London were important in this finding; London has low mortality from coronary heart disease and, in the past, had low neonatal but high postneonatal mortality. Possible reasons for this are examined later, in chapter 10. As a further exploration the 212 local authority groups were ordered according to the neonatal mortality rates during 1911–25 and divided into five groups according to the level of mortality.[23] Neonatal mortality rose from 30 per 1000 births in group 1 to 44 in group 5. Five groups with increasing postneonatal mortality were derived in the same way, mortality rising from 32 per 1000 in group 1 to 73 in group 5. In this way the relationship of neonatal and postneonatal mortality to adult mortality could be examined within a grid of 25 cells (table1.1). Areas with low neonatal but high postneonatal mortality were mainly in London, although they included the towns of Chester and Great Yarmouth. Areas with high neonatal but low postneonatal mortalities were scattered through the north and west, including the rural areas of Anglesey, Northumberland, and Staffordshire.

The table compares death rates from stroke, coronary heart disease, and chronic bronchitis. Within any of the five bands of postneonatal mortality, standardised mortality ratios for stroke increase sharply with increasing

TABLE 1.1—*Standardised mortality ratios from stroke, coronary heart disease, and chronic bronchitis (ages 35–74, both sexes, 1968–78) in the 212 areas of England and Wales grouped by neonatal and postneonatal mortality (1911–25)*

		Postneonatal mortality				
		1 (lowest)	2	3	4	5 (highest)
Neonatal mortality						
	1 (lowest)	85	81	79	78	79
	2	86	90	98	74	76
Stroke	3	102	100	104	104	104
	4	–	108	110	115	117
	5 (highest)	124	–	121	123	117
	1 (lowest)	84	89	91	88	98
Coronary	2	85	93	95	88	91
heart	3	86	94	99	106	113
disease	4	–	98	109	111	115
	5 (highest)	83	–	114	119	116
	1 (lowest)	67	78	106	115	161
	2	64	84	85	104	126
Chronic	3	69	65	89	88	151
bronchitis	4	–	91	99	120	142
	5 (highest)	41	–	108	123	144

neonatal mortality. There is no independent trend in stroke mortality with postneonatal mortality. Mortality from coronary heart disease has similar but separate trends with neonatal and postneonatal mortality. Mortality from chronic bronchitis shows a steep increase with increasing postneonatal mortality, but no independent trend with neonatal mortality.

Seventy years ago most neonatal deaths occurred within a week of birth, and depended on adverse intrauterine rather than postnatal influences.[24] Eighty per cent of such deaths were certified to be the result of "congenital" causes, which also correlate geographically with stroke and coronary heart disease. The link between neonatal mortality and cardiovascular disease therefore suggests that early influences predisposing to cardiovascular disease act during prenatal life. Postneonatal deaths were the result of respiratory infection, diarrhoea, and other infections, reflecting inadequate housing, overcrowding, and other adverse influences in the environment after birth. The association between chronic bronchitis and respiratory infection in infancy is discussed in chapter 7.

Maternal nutrition and health

The relationship between cardiovascular disease and the intrauterine environment can be explored further by examining maternal mortality. In Britain maternal mortality remained at a disturbingly high level from the late nineteenth century until the mid-1930s.[25] "A deep, dark and continuous stream of mortality." In the early part of this century the geographical distribution of maternal mortality in Britain was similar to that of neonatal mortality.[26]

> Maternal mortality tends to be highest in rural, sparsely populated counties, and in industrial districts, notably those associated with the textile industries in Lancashire and Yorkshire, and with coal mining; and tends to be lowest in the South of England, in districts in and around London, and in certain large towns, such as Birmingham, Manchester and Liverpool.

Two early reports analysed the causes of maternal mortality,[26 27] grouping deaths into those caused by puerperal fever (around 40%) and those caused by "other complications of pregnancy and parturition". Most of these "other" deaths resulted from toxaemia, haemorrhage, or accidents of childbirth.

Fig 1.5 shows that the geographical distribution of stroke correlates closely with past maternal deaths from these "other causes":[28] the correlation coefficient is 0·65. The relationship occurs in both sexes and is specific. Among other causes of death, only coronary heart disease correlates as closely with past maternal mortality. As expected from table 1.1, maternal mortality is unrelated to chronic bronchitis.

In his analysis of infant mortality in Britain, Woolf[22] stated that much of the variation in neonatal mortality depended on variations in poverty, as measured by the percentage of unemployed men in the lower socioeconomic groups. He attributed this to the adverse effects of poverty on maternal nutrition and lactation. Campbell's[26 29] earlier analyses had also identified poor health and physique of mothers as a major cause of maternal mortality. She attributed them to poor nutrition, rickets in infancy, and industrial employment of girls. Baird[30 31] also related the large geographical differences in perinatal mortality in Britain to differences in the physique and health of women. He concluded that the poor living standards which accompanied industrialisation or economic depression adversely affected the development of young girls, and impaired their subsequent reproductive efficiency.

HYPOTHESIS

An interpretation of the analyses described here is that poor nutrition, health, and development among girls and young women is the origin of high death rates from cardiovascular disease in the next generation. It prejudices the ability of mothers to nourish their babies *in utero* and during infancy. The fetus responds to undernutrition with permanent changes in its physiology and metabolism, and these lead to coronary heart disease and stroke in adult life.

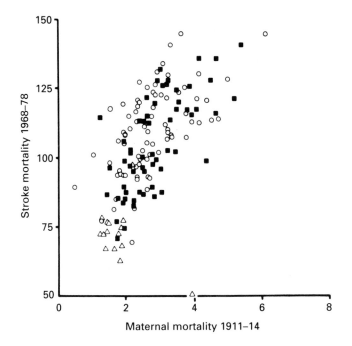

FIG 1.5—*Standardised mortality ratios for stroke in men and women aged 55–74 years during 1968–78, and maternal mortality (per 1000) from "other causes" (see text) during 1911–14.*

Migrants

If the environment *in utero* and during infancy influences the development of cardiovascular disease, a person's risk of that disease will be related to his or her place of birth. This can be explored by examining disease rates in people who migrate from their place of birth, because the effects of the environment in early life can be distinguished from that encountered later on. In England and Wales, where variations in maternal and neonatal mortality suggest differences in maternal nutrition from place to place, disease in migrants can be analysed using data from death certificates. Place of birth is recorded on death certificates, although it is not routinely coded. For a trial period during 1969–72, however, the Office of Population Censuses and Surveys (OPCS) did code the place of birth. During this time there were almost two million deaths in England and Wales among people who had been born there. Of these people half had migrated to another part of the country during their lives.

Using these data, Osmond[32][33] related numbers of deaths from coronary heart disease and stroke, expressed as a proportion of all deaths, to place of birth and place of death. The results showed that a person's risk of dying from coronary heart disease or stroke was predicted by place of birth, independent of place of death. Part of the increased risk among people born in many northern counties and industrial towns, and in Wales, persisted whether or not they had moved to other areas of the country. The low risk of cardiovascular disease, especially stroke, among people born in and around London went with them when they moved.

The results of this study conflicted with the conclusions of two small studies of coronary heart disease and blood pressure in middle aged men who migrated within Britain.[34][35] In these studies the occurrence of coronary heart disease, of which there were 43 episodes, was unrelated to place of birth; blood pressure among men who migrated from the north to the south of England was lower than that of men who remained in the north. These findings are, however, confounded by birthweight. The average birthweight of men who migrate is higher than that of men who remain in the area where they were born,[36] and men with higher birthweight have lower blood pressure (see chapter 4). Evidence from migrant studies is necessarily inconclusive because people who migrate from the place where they were born differ from those who remain. The balance of evidence is, however, consistent with the hypothesis that the intrauterine environment influences cardiovascular disease.

Summary

The suggestion that events in childhood influence the pathogenesis of cardiovascular disease is not new. The implication of the geographical studies described in this chapter is, however, that the search for environmental causes of cardiovascular disease should not focus on the environment of children, their diets, homes, and illnesses, but rather should focus on babies, for whom mothers are the dominant environmental influence. This is a new point of departure for cardiovascular research.

1 Pisa Z, Uemura K. Trends of mortality from ischaemic heart disease and other cardiovascular diseases in 27 countries, 1968–1977. *World Health Stat Q* 1982;**35**: 11–47.

2 Greaves JP, Hollingsworth DF. Trends in food consumption in the United Kingdom. *World Rev Nutr Diet* 1966;**6**:34–89.

3 Southgate DAT, Bingham S, Robertson J. Dietary fibre in the British diet. *Nature* 1978; **274**:51–2.

4 Barker DJP, Osmond C. Diet and coronary heart disease in England and Wales during and after the second world war. *J Epidemiol Community Health* 1986;**40**:37–44.

5 Office of Population Censuses and Surveys. *Registrar General's statistical review of England and Wales. Part 1. Tables, medical.* London: HMSO, 1911 *et seq.*

6 Ryle JA, Russell WT. The natural history of coronary disease. A clinical and epidemiological study. *Br Heart J* 1949;**11**:370–89.

7 Morris JN. Recent history of coronary disease. *Lancet* 1951;**i**:1–7.

8 Gardner MJ, Crawford MD, Morris JN. Patterns of mortality in middle and early old age in the county boroughs of England and Wales. *Br J Prev Soc Med* 1969;**23**: 133–40.

9 *Resistrar General's decennial supplement, occupational mortality, England and Wales 1970–72.* London: HMSO, 1978.

10 Keys A. *Seven countries.* Cambridge, MA: Harvard University Press, 1980.

11 Rose G, Marmot MG. Social class and coronary heart disease. *Br Heart J* 1981;**45**: 13–19.

12 Rose G. Sick individuals and sick populations. *Int J Epidemiol* 1985;**14**:32–8.

13 Barker DJP, Osmond C. Infant mortality, childhood nutrition, and ischaemic heart disease in England and Wales. *Lancet* 1986;**i**:1077–81.

14 Gardner MJ, Winter PD, Barker DJP. *Atlas of mortality from selected diseases in England and Wales 1968–78.* Chichester: Wiley, 1984.

15 Office of Population Censuses and Surveys. *The dietary and nutritional survey of British adults.* London: HMSO, 1990.

16 Forsdahl A. Are poor living conditions in childhood and adolescence an important risk factor for arteriosclerotic heart disease? *Br J Prev Soc Med* 1977;**31**:91–5.

17 Notkola V. *Living conditions in childhood and coronary heart disease in adulthood.* Helsinki: Finnish Society of Sciences and Letters, 1985.

18 Buck C, Simpson H. Infant diarrhoea and subsequent mortality from heart disease and cancer. *J Epidemiol Community Health* 1982;**36**:27–30.

19 Rose G. Familial patterns in ischaemic heart disease. *Br J Prev Soc Med* 1964;**18**:75–80.

20 Marmot MG, Shipley MH, Rose G. Inequalities in death – specific explanations of a general pattern? *Lancet* 1984;**i**:1003–6.

21 Hinkle LE. Coronary heart disease and sudden death in actively employed American men. *Bull NY Acad Med* 1973;**49**:467–74.

22 Woolf B. Studies on infant mortality: part II, social aetiology of stillbirths and infant deaths in county boroughs of England and Wales. *Br J Social Med* 1947;**1**:73–125.

23 Barker DJP, Osmond C, Law CM. The intrauterine and early postnatal origins of cardiovascular disease and chronic bronchitis. *J Epidemiol Community Health* 1989; **43**:237–40.

24 Local Government Board. *Thirty-ninth annual report 1909–10. Supplement on infant and child mortality.* London: HMSO, 1910.

25 Loudon I. Deaths in childhood from the eighteenth century to 1935. *Medical History* 1986;**30**:1–41.

26 Campbell JM. *Maternal mortality.* London: HMSO, 1924. (Ministry of Health Reports on Public Health and Medical Subjects, No. 25.)

27 Local Government Board. *Forty-fourth annual report 1914–15. Supplement on Maternal mortality in connection with childbearing.* London: HMSO, 1916.

28 Barker DJP, Osmond C. Death rates from stroke in England and Wales predicted from past maternal mortality. *BMJ* 1987;**295**:83–6.

29 Campbell JM, Cameron D, Jones DM. *High maternal mortality in certain areas.* London: HMSO, 1932. (Ministry of Health Reports on Public Health and Medical Subjects, No. 68.)

30 Baird D. Social factors in obstetrics. *Lancet* 1949;**i**:1079–83.

31 Baird D. Environment and reproduction. *Br J Obstet Gynaecol* 1980;**87**:1057–67.

32 Osmond C, Slattery JM, Barker DJP. Mortality by place of birth. In: *Mortality and geography: a review in the mid 1980s. OPCS Series DS No 9.* London: HMSO, 1990: chapter 8.

33 Osmond C, Barker DJP, Slattery JM. Risk of death from cardiovascular disease and chronic bronchitis determined by place of birth in England and Wales. *J Epidemiol Community Health* 1990;**44**:139–41.

34 Elford J, Phillips AN, Thomson AG, Shaper AG. Migration and geographic variations in ischaemic heart disease in Great Britain. *Lancet* 1989;**i**:343–6.
35 Elford J, Phillips AN, Thomson AG, Shaper AG. Migration and geographic variations in blood pressure in Britain. *BMJ* 1990;**300**:291–5.
36 Martyn CN, Barker DJP, Osmond C. Selective migration by birthweight. *J Epidemiol Community Health* 1993;**47**:76.

2: Programming the baby

The findings described in chapter 1 led to the hypothesis that undernutrition *in utero* and during infancy permanently changes the body's structure, physiology, and metabolism, and leads to coronary heart disease and stroke in adult life. The principle that the nutritional, hormonal, and metabolic environment afforded by the mother may permanently "program" the structure and physiology of her offspring was established long ago. Lucas[1] proposed the term "programming" to describe the process whereby a stimulus or insult, at a critical period of development, has lasting or lifelong significance. This chapter describes the extensive observations on programming in animals that allow us to understand the observations now being made in humans.

Animal studies have established four principles which underlie programming. First, undernutrition in early life has permanent effects. Second, undernutrition has different effects at different times in early life. Third, rapidly growing fetuses and neonates are more vulnerable to undernutrition. Fourth, the permanent effects of undernutrition include reduced cell numbers, altered organ structure, and resetting of hormonal axes.

Sensitive periods in development

One of the best examples of the phenomenon known as *programming* is the lifelong effect of early exposure to sex hormones on sexual physiology. A female rat injected with testosterone propionate on day five after birth develops normally until puberty, but fails to ovulate or show normal patterns of female sexual behaviour thereafter.[2] Pituitary and ovarian function are normal, but the release of gonadotrophin by the hypothalamus has been irreversibly altered from the cyclical female pattern of release to the tonic male pattern. If the same injection of testosterone is given when the animal is 20 days old, it has no effect. Thus there is a critical time at which the animal's sexual physiology is sensitive and can be permanently changed.

Numerous animal experiments such as this have shown that hormones, undernutrition, and other influences that affect development during sensitive periods of early life permanently program the structure and physiology of the body's tissues and systems.[2-11] The body is most susceptible to programming when it is growing rapidly.[12] During the first two months of life, the embryonic period, the human differentiates but does not grow rapidly. Thereafter, in the fetal period, it attains its highest growth rate.

14

Growth slows in late gestation and throughout childhood. The high growth rates of the fetus compared with the child are largely the result of cell replication. The proportion of cells that are dividing becomes progressively less as the fetus becomes older, so that few new nerve or muscle cells, for example, appear after 30 weeks of gestation.[13] The concept of sensitive periods in early life is familiar from experiments in which animals have been imprinted to behave abnormally. Lorenz[14] showed that newly hatched goslings could be imprinted to behave as if a dog were their mother—if the first moving object they saw after hatching was a dog. Long ago Pliny described "a goose which followed Lacydes as faithfully as a dog" and Reginald of Durham wrote of eider-ducks which followed humans.

A remarkable example of programming is the effect of temperature on the sex of reptiles. If the eggs of the American alligator are incubated at 30°C all the offspring are female. If they are incubated at 33°C all the offspring are male. At temperatures between 30 and 33°C there are varying proportions of females and males. It is believed that the fundamental sex is female, and a transcription factor is required to divert growth along a male pathway. Instead of the transcription factor being controlled genetically, by a sex chromosome, it depends on the environment, specifically temperature. The temperature at which the eggs are incubated also determines postnatal growth rates, skin pigmentation, and the animal's preferred temperature— alligators will seek out an environment that has the same temperature as the one in which they were hatched.[15] It is postulated that one of the mechanisms controlling the long term effects of incubation temperature is the pulsatile release of hormones from the hypothalamus.[16]

In some animals, such as the pig, cell numbers increase most rapidly after birth rather than before, and the animal can therefore recover from undernutrition *in utero*. Humans, however, accomplish a greater proportion of their growth before birth than pigs, and the effects of intrauterine growth failure are more severe.[17] It has been calculated that the fertilised human ovum goes through some 42 rounds of cell division before birth.[18] After birth only a further five cycles of division are needed. Tissues develop in a predetermined sequence from conception to maturity,[19] with different organs and tissues undergoing periods of rapid cell division, and therefore being in sensitive periods, at different times. The renal nephrons, for example, are laid down during the last trimester of pregnancy whereas the pancreatic β cells continue to differentiate during infancy.[20 21]

Growth and form of the body

The pigs in fig 2.1 are littermates. However, they have been reared on different diets with the result that two of them are small and have different body proportions. Slowing of growth is a major adaptation to undernutrition, because if the smallest pig, given an inferior diet, had maintained the same growth trajectory as the largest it would have perished.

15

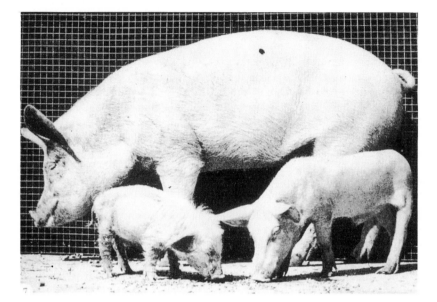

FIG 2.1—*Three pigs from the same litter reared on different diets.*

Numerous experiments on animals, including rats, mice, sheep, and pigs, have shown that, when the protein or calorie intake of the mother during pregnancy and lactation is lowered, the offspring are smaller than they would otherwise have been.[17 22-31] In general, the earlier in the life of an animal that undernutrition occurs, the more likely it is to have permanent effects on body weight and length.[30] Figs 2.2 and 2.3 show the results of an experiment carried out by Widdowson and McCance[32] 30 years ago. Rats who were undernourished from three to six weeks after birth, that is, immediately after weaning, lost weight. On resumption of full feeding at six weeks, they failed to return to the growth trajectory of the controls and remained permanently small (fig 2.2). By contrast, rats who were not undernourished until 9–12 weeks after birth regained their growth trajectory when full feeding was resumed, and continued to grow normally (fig 2.3).

Early in fetal life growth is regulated by the supply of nutrients and oxygen. At some point before birth, or shortly after in some species, growth begins to "track". Animals who are small in relation to others of the same age remain small, and vice versa. In humans tracking is demonstrated by the way in which infants grow along centile curves.[30] Once tracking is established it is no longer possible to make animals grow faster by offering them unlimited food. Their rate of growth has become "set", homoeostatically controlled by feedback systems. After a period of undernutrition, they will regain their expected size. If they consume excess food they will merely become fat.

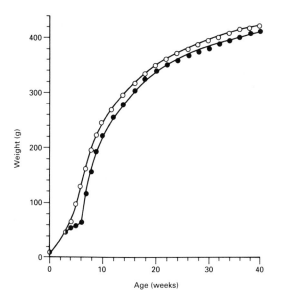

FIG 2.2—*Rats undernourished from three to six weeks after birth remain permanently small.*

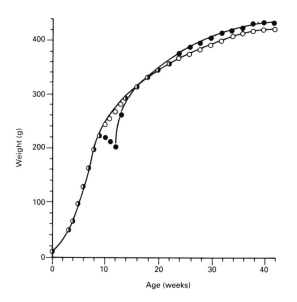

FIG 2.3—*The growth of rats undernourished from nine to 12 weeks after birth catches up.*

17

In early intrauterine life undernutrition tends to produce small but normally proportioned animals, such as the "runt" pig, whereas at later stages of development it leads to selective organ damage.[30] During periods of undernutrition those tissues whose maturity is more advanced have a greater priority for growth and may continue to grow at the expense of other tissues.[33] For example, when rats are undernourished immediately after weaning, the weight of the brain and skeletal muscle is unaffected but the weight of the liver, kidney, and thymus is permanently reduced. When, however, undernutrition is delayed until 42 days after birth only the thymus is affected.

If growth is restricted by a reduced blood supply, rather than through undernutrition, the results are similar. If, for example, the artery supplying one horn of the rat's uterus is occluded in late gestation, the brain is spared but growth of the liver is disproportionately retarded. In general both undernutrition and uteroplacental ischaemia have the same effects on proportionate fetal growth if they occur at the same time.[34 35] The timing of the insult is the factor that determines which tissues and systems are damaged, and hence the disproportion in size and function. The pattern of disproportion will also be influenced by the relative sensitivity of different organs. Some aspects of maturation, such as the growth of the thymus, are markedly influenced by nutrition, whereas others, such as the growth of the eye, are less sensitive.[36] The eye grows with chronological age and its development is less "plastic" than that of most other tissues.

The way in which an animal's body proportions are modified by undernutrition is also related to its growth trajectory. If rats are undernourished for a brief three week period after weaning, those who were previously growing rapidly have different body compositions from those who were growing slowly—even if both groups of animals have the same final body weight. The bones of the fast growing rats are longer and the testes heavier, but the livers, spleens, and small intestines are lighter.[32] Similarly, in sheep the response of the fetus to maternal undernutrition in late pregnancy depends on its growth rate.[37] Slow growing fetuses are unaffected whereas the growth of rapidly growing fetuses ceases abruptly (fig 2.4). One possible explanation is that slowly growing fetuses have previously encountered undernutrition, in early pregnancy, and adapted to it by recruiting more placentomes. This protects them from restricted nutrition in later gestation. Again the size of the lambs at birth is similar although their body compositions differ. Placental enlargement as an adaptation to undernutrition is discussed further in chapter 9. In humans, the growth trajectory of boys is more rapid than that of girls from early in embryonic life. Boys are therefore more vulnerable to undernutrition and this could explain their higher rates of coronary heart disease (chapter 3).

The nature of the undernutrition, as well as its timing, severity, and the fetal growth trajectory, may influence body proportions. Pigs reared on

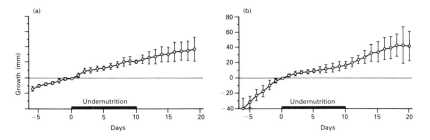

FIG 2.4—*Slow growing fetal lambs are unaffected by undernutrition (a) but the growth of rapidly growing fetuses slows (b).*

very small amounts of good quality diet become small and thin. Those reared on the same diet but with unlimited amounts of carbohydrate or fat become somewhat larger. The brains of both groups of animals are disproportionately large, the bones continue to grow, whereas muscles scarcely grow at all, and the ovaries become cystic. The extra growth ocurring as a result of the "protein sparing effect" of unlimited energy leads to exaggerated enlargement of the penis and vulva.[30 33 38]

Small human babies are either proportionate, that is, "perfect miniatures", or disproportionate. Consistent with the findings in animals, the symmetrically small baby is thought to originate through undernutrition in early gestation. The disproportionate baby is thought to result from undernutrition in later gestation. In other words, undernutrition in early gestation affects body size permanently, whereas undernutrition in late gestation has profound effects on body form. The long term consequences of different kinds of disproportion at birth are a recurring theme of this book and are introduced in chapter 3.

The mechanisms which underlie programming

The many permanent changes that are now known to be induced by undernutrition and other adverse influences in early life raise the question of how the memory of these events is stored and later expressed. Lucas has postulated three cellular mechanisms.[1] First, the nutrient environment may permanently alter gene expression;[39] for example, permanent changes in activity of HMG-CoA reductase and other enzymes induced in animal experiments are described in this chapter.

Second, early nutrition may permanently reduce cell numbers. The small but normally proportioned rat produced by undernutrition before weaning has been shown to have fewer cells in its organs and tissues.[3 24 27] Winick and colleagues[40] suggested that for this reason the animal does not regain its full size when adequately nourished after weaning. They argued that, as cell division cannot be restarted after the period of rapid division has come to an end, cell numbers limit ultimate body size. Growth retarded human babies have reduced numbers of cells in their organs[41] and in some instances these reduced numbers of cells can be directly linked to limitations of function. For example, reduced numbers of pancreatic β cells may limit insulin secretion and reduced size of the airways may limit respiratory function.

The third cellular mechanism of programming may be the selection of clones of cells. Atopic disease, for example, is characterised by an altered balance of the Th1 and Th2 lymphocyte subtypes. It has been suggested that this imbalance results from impairment of thymic development in late fetal life.[42]

In addition to cellular mechanisms, the memory of early undernutrition may persist through permanent changes in organ structure. Hoet and colleagues have shown that, in the rat, protein deficiency not only lowers β cell mass in the pancreas but reduces the vascularisation of the islets— which may further impair insulin secretion.[43]

Undernutrition may also effect permanent changes through intermediary mechanisms; the possible role of hormones as intermediaries is a recurring theme of this book. Sensitivity to hormones may be programmed by the setting of cell receptors—structures in the cell membrane which convey the signal mediated by the hormone into the cell. Experiments suggest that membrane receptors are plastic during critical periods of maturation, and their structure may be permanently altered. Exposure to a normal concentration of hormone seems to promote receptor development, whereas exposure to other hormones that are sufficiently similar to bind to the receptor may reduce the receptor response permanently.[44 45] A single dose of gonadotrophin hormone, which is similar in structure to thyroid-stimulating hormone (TSH), permanently changes the TSH receptors and reduces the responsiveness of the thyroid to TSH, with consequent reduction in thyroxine levels.[46]

Imprinting of the hypothalamus may determine the long term pattern of release of pituitary hormones. The cyclical release of gonadotrophins is known to be determined in this way (see page 28). Hypothalamic imprinting is suspected of underlying the long term effects of incubation temperature in reptiles, and it may prove an important mechanism in the causation of human disease.

Summary

Undernutrition and other adverse influences arising in fetal life or immediately after birth have a permanent effect on the body's structure, physiology, and metabolism. The specific effects of undernutrition depend on the time in development at which it occurs. In early gestation undernutrition reduces body size permanently, whereas in late gestation it has profound effects on body form without necessarily reducing body size. Rapidly growing fetuses and neonates are more vulnerable to undernutrition. The effects include altered gene expression, reduced cell numbers, imbalance between cell types, altered organ structure, the pattern of hormonal release, and setting of hormonal responses.

The remainder of this chapter reviews what is known about the long term effects of early undernutrition on the different tissues and systems of the body. No review has been published recently, and the authors hope that it will prove useful as a source of reference to others working in this field. The general reader should turn to chapter 3.

Maturation and ageing

The offspring of rats, pigs, and guinea pigs which are undernourished before birth stop growing at the normal chronological age and are therefore small as adults. Animals undernourished after birth, however, delay development and continue to grow beyond the normal age. In delaying development, and sexual maturation, these animals resemble humans in undernourished communities in the developing world.[30] Although some aspects of sexual maturation may be postponed by undernutrition, others seem to be protected. The experiments on pigs already cited suggest that development of the external genitalia is protected even during intense undernutrition.[33]

In rats, undernutrition *in utero* and up to weaning at three weeks after birth is followed in middle age by a more rapid progression of albuminuria and an increased activity of enzymes associated with ageing.[28] In the mouse, undernutrition during the last week of gestation leads to a reduction in peak haemoglobin and a more rapid decline in haemoglobin in later life.[47] Such findings suggest that perinatal undernutrition may be linked to more rapid ageing, which contrasts with the results of numerous experiments showing that reduced nutrient intake after weaning reduces the rate of growth, prolongs the period of growth, postpones sexual maturation, and prolongs lifespan.[48-53]

A recent theory of ageing suggests that, in terms of evolutionary benefit, there is a trade off between allocation of energy to either reproduction or repair of somatic damage. Such damage necessarily occurs as a result of extrinsic and intrinsic insults throughout life, and increases the rate of ageing. Species in which the young are exposed to high early mortality, for example, from predators, may benefit from more prolific reproduction at the expense of more prolonged survival of individuals.[54] It is postulated that fetal undernutrition leads not only to an immediate reduction in growth rate but to reduced expression of genes responsible for somatic repair. Under this hypothesis the fetus is adapting to an adverse environment, and a perceived reduced life expectancy, by diverting resources to reproduction. It thus becomes more vulnerable to somatic damage, which manifests in more rapid ageing through failure to sustain mitosis and to produce specific proteins.

OBESITY

Animal experiments show that early overnutrition may have permanent effects on body weight, and carbohydrate and lipid metabolism.[55-58] People who become obese during childhood tend to remain fat in adult life.[59] Paradoxically, however, early starvation may also be followed by adult obesity. Among men born during the Dutch Hunger Winter of 1944–1945, those exposed to famine in the first half of gestation became obese as adults.[60 61] It is thought that in early gestation hypothalamic control of appetite becomes set in relation to body size.[12 62] An inappropriate setting of the hypothalamus could have led to the obesity of the men exposed to famine *in utero*.

In contrast to the men exposed to famine in the first half of gestation, those who starved during late gestation and the first month after birth remained thin.[61] It has been suggested that the numbers of adipocytes—fat storing cells—are established in late gestation and early infancy. Rats given a reduced calorie intake during suckling have been found to have a permanently decreased number of adipocytes.[63 64] However, observations on baboons are not consistent with this, and suggest that infant nutrition influences cell size rather than cell numbers.[58] The importance of early programming of adipocyte numbers in the development of human obesity remains unresolved.

ORGAN GROWTH

Brain—The growth of the brain occurs in two phases. Multiplication of neuronal and glial cells is followed by the outgrowth of dendrons and axons. The extensive literature on the long term consequences of nutritional, hormonal, and other environmental influences on brain growth has been brought together in a number of recent reviews.[65-68]

There is considerable evidence that early undernutrition adversely affects neurological, cognitive, and emotional development. As with other tissues, undernutrition generally affects those parts of the brain that are undergoing rapid differentiation at the time, even though the brain tends to be "spared" in relation to other organs.[5 11 69 70] Hormone concentrations influence brain development. Corticosteroids affect the rate of brain cell acquisition whereas thyroid hormones affect the timing of periods of rapid brain cell division. Gonadal hormones control the development of sexual physiology and behaviour.

Studies of visual development provide some of the best known observations on the importance of environmental stimulation in brain development.[71 72] Temporary closure of the lids of one eye in kittens, for example, causes neurons in the visual cortex to become unresponsive to signals through the deprived eye, which is blind.

Lucas[73] has demonstrated programming in humans in studies of preterm infants randomly assigned to either a standard formula for term infants or a nutrient-enriched formula. Infants assigned to the standard formula, for only a few weeks after birth, had major deficiencies in developmental scores at 18 months of age. The deficiencies were particularly marked in motor development where the deficit was of the order of one standard deviation. The greatest deficiencies were seen in children who were small for gestation, that is, already undernourished at birth. Preliminary findings of a parallel study suggest that breast milk promotes cognitive development, protects against allergy, but restricts linear growth.[74] Although the findings in these remarkable studies cannot necessarily be generalised to normal infants, born at term, they provide experimental support for the thesis that nutritional programming during sensitive periods in early life influences long term health and development.

Lung—In animals, a fetus deprived of calories or oxygen may develop pulmonary hypoplasia, defined by a reduction in the ratio of lung weight to body weight or a reduction in total lung DNA.[75-79] In the rat, interference with fetal growth can induce lung changes that resemble human emphysema, with persisting reduction in elastin and collagen, enlargement of airspaces, and a loss of elastic recoil.[80-84]

The timing of undernutrition determines whether its effects are permanent. In guinea pigs, whose alveolar development is largely completed before birth,[85] fetal undernutrition permanently changes alveolar morphology, whereas the changes induced by postnatal undernutrition are reversible.[86 87] In rats, whose lungs undergo a period of rapid cell replication between four and 13 days after birth,[88 89] permanent changes in alveolar structure can be induced by protein or calorie restriction in early postnatal life,[83] whereas changes induced after weaning may be reversible.[82 87]

In humans airway division down the the level of the terminal bronchioles is completed by week 16 of gestation.[90] Around half of the adult number of alveoli are present at birth, and cell multiplication is almost complete by two years of age (see chapter 7, p. 101). Pulmonary hypoplasia is common *post mortem*, being found in 14% of perinatal postmortem examinations and in 27% of late spontaneous abortions in one study.[91]

Physical influences are important in the regulation of lung growth.[92] An adequate amount of fluid within the airways appears to be necessary. In animals, reducing the volume of amniotic fluid[93-95] or draining lung fluid from the airways[96 97] leads to pulmonary hypoplasia. Similarly, in humans, oligohydramnios is associated with lung hypoplasia and narrow airways.[91 98] The earlier the onset of the reduction in amniotic fluid volume, the more severe the degree of lung hypoplasia.[99 100] A congenital diaphragmatic hernia allows abdominal contents to encroach on the intrathoracic space and is associated with a reduction in the number of airway branches.[101 102] The growing chest wall is thought to provide a "stretch" stimulus for growth of the underlying lung.[103] Abnormal chest wall growth, as a result of either compression in association with oligohydramnios[94 103] or skeletal deformity in kyphoscoliosis, impairs lung development.[104 105]

Kidney—In the rat, restriction of the mother's protein intake leads to smaller kidneys, with fewer and less differentiated glomeruli and collecting tubules.[106] It has recently been shown that rats born to mothers who had low protein intakes before and during pregnancy have persistently raised blood pressure.[107] It is not known whether or not the raised blood pressure is mediated through the kidney. In humans, 60% of the normal complement of nephrons develop during the last trimester and development of the kidney ceases around week 35.[21 108] Babies with disproportionate growth retardation, whose bodies are relatively small in relation to their heads, have a markedly reduced number of nephrons at birth. This pattern of disproportion, which is thought to be a consequence of impaired development in the last trimester, is followed by raised blood pressure in adult life (see chapter 4).

Intestine—In the rat the intestine develops rapidly in late gestation, and low maternal protein intake at this time leads to marked changes in structure, especially in the small intestine. The villi are fewer and less well differentiated.[109] In the same experiments liver structure was not affected. This is interesting because there has been speculation that abnormalities in lipid metabolism may derive from an imbalance between intestinal and hepatic function.

METABOLISM

Lipid metabolism—Cholesterol is an essential component of cell membranes and is a metabolic precursor of steroid hormones. It is synthesised *de novo* in the body and is also absorbed from the diet. With a varying supply of dietary cholesterol, the body maintains tissue concentrations by a balance between synthesis, controlled by the enzyme 3-hydroxy-3-methylglutaryl-coenzyme A reductase (HMG-CoA reductase), and excretion, mainly in the bile after conversion to bile acids.[110]

There has been considerable speculation that the high cholesterol content and saturated fat content of human milk may program lipid metabolism throughout life and thereby influence the risk of cardiovascular disease. The results of early experiments gave some support to this hypothesis because animals suckled on low cholesterol-containing milk were found to have raised serum cholesterol concentrations subsequently, by reason of high activity of HMG-CoA reductase in the liver.[111 112] However, the results of other experiments and follow up studies of infants into childhood have failed to support the hypothesis.[110] The concentration of cholesterol in infants' food seems to have no more than a transient effect on serum cholesterol concentrations.[113-115]

Although cholesterol intake in infancy may not be important in the long term, animal experiments have unequivocally demonstrated that interference with cholesterol metabolism during development, by either changing the composition of the diet or giving cholestyramine, which increases cholesterol excretion, has permanent effects. Manipulations during gestation up regulate cholesterol synthesis,[110 116] whereas manipulations after birth permanently change the body's capacity to excrete cholesterol in bile. The system of bile acid synthesis and excretion may be too immature in fetal life to be programmed.[117] When given to newborn guinea pigs, cholestyramine reduces the elevation of cholesterol in response to a dietary cholesterol challenge by increasing bile acid excretion.[114 118 119]

The age at which an animal is weaned also appears to have a long lasting influence on metabolism.[120-122] Weaning onto solid food entails a sharp fall in fat intake and a rise in carbohydrate intake. Rats that are prematurely weaned have a raised serum cholesterol in later life, which only becomes apparent after seven months.[121 123] Rats given a low protein diet after weaning have a significantly lower bile flow and bile acid secretion.[124]

Mott and Lewis's experiments on baboons have shown that breast feeding leads to a higher low density lipoprotein cholesterol to high density lipoprotein cholesterol ratio in later life than is found in formula fed baboons.[10 125-127] As, in humans, a high ratio is linked to coronary heart disease, this could suggest that breast feeding is associated with an unfavourable outcome. Another interpretation, however, is that breast fed animals use cholesterol more efficiently, having an increased absorption and reduced turnover. Other experiments in baboons have suggested that it is not the ingested cholesterol which permanently changes lipid metabolism but the hormones or growth factors contained in breast milk. Thyroid hormone may be important, resetting thyroid homoeostasis and hence mediating sustained differences in cholesterol and bile acid metabolism.[10 128-130]

In the human infant, serum cholesterol concentration is related to day to day intake of cholesterol and saturated fat.[131-134] From around the age of six months, serum cholesterol concentrations tend to "track" so that children maintain their rank order by concentration through childhood.[135 136] Two recent studies suggest that raised serum cholesterol concentrations in humans may be programmed through failure of development of the liver in late gestation and by prolonged breast feeding.[137 138] These studies are discussed in chapter 5.

Protein metabolism—Studies of protein metabolism in both humans and rats suggest that the mother's intake of protein may program nitrogen metabolism in her children.[139 140] Children whose mothers had a low protein intake in pregnancy were found to excrete an unusually high proportion of their absorbed nitrogen.

ENDOCRINE

Insulin—This hormone is of central importance to fetal growth and metabolism, and has been intensively studied in both fetal animals and humans.[141] It stimulates growth by increasing the mitotic drive and nutrient availability for cell proliferation. It increases the utilisation of glucose and reduces the catabolism of amino acids. It responds to nutrient levels and acts as a signal of nutrient sufficiency, ensuring that fetal growth rates are commensurate with the nutrient supply.[142] The pancreatic β cells seem highly sensitive to dietary protein. In the rat a low protein diet during pregnancy reduces the β cell mass and profoundly reduces islet vascularisation.[43] A low protein diet, given for only three weeks after weaning, permanently impairs the insulin response to glucose.[8] In the mouse undernutrition during lactation also permanently lowers serum insulin concentrations.[29] There is evidence from studies of rats and dogs that protein deficiency after weaning makes the animals insulin resistant.[143 144]

Remarkable experiments by van Assche and Aerts[145] have shown that changes in the glucose concentrations to which a fetus is exposed produce effects through several generations, mimicking genetic transmission. Pregnant rats were made mildly diabetic by injection of streptozocin on the day of mating. Their female offspring developed gestational diabetes when they became pregnant and, in turn, their offspring developed islet cell hyperplasia β-cell degradation, and disordered glucose metabolism as adults. The changes in the third generation were independent of the origins of the father.

Whereas in the human fetus raised plasma glucose concentrations, caused by gestational diabetes, lead to hyperinsulinaemia, the undernourished, growth retarded fetus may have reduced numbers of β cells and reduced insulin secretion.[146 147] The links between insulin deficiency and resistance, acquired *in utero*, and non-insulin dependent diabetes in later life are discussed in chapter 6.

Growth hormone—In late gestation growth hormone assumes increasing importance in driving fetal growth. Babies with growth hormone deficiency are relatively short at birth, although of normal weight.[148] Limited evidence suggests that growth hormone secretion may be permanently influenced by events in early life. In particular, studies in rats have suggested that maternal dietary restriction during gestation and lactation may permanently reduce growth hormone secretion in the offspring.[149 150]

Insulin-like growth factor I (IGF-I) is an important regulator of fetal growth, and is itself regulated by nutrition and growth hormone.[148] Transient starvation lowers fetal IGF-I concentrations, which are rapidly restored by replacement of glucose or insulin.[151 152] Growth retarded fetal sheep, however, have low circulating IGF-I concentrations which fail to increase in response to restoration of glucose supply. This suggests that chronic undernutrition permanently reduces IGF-I production.[153]

In humans the growth retarded fetus who is not growth hormone deficient, but who shows slow postnatal growth, has elevated growth hormone concentrations and reduced IGF-I concentrations.[154-156] These babies may therefore be resistant to growth hormone. Support for this conclusion comes from recent findings in children in England[157] and India (unpublished): growth hormone concentrations were found to be highest in children who had the lowest birthweight, irrespective of current size.

Cortisol—In contrast to insulin, which has an important role in tissue accretion during fetal life, the main effects of cortisol are on cell differentiation.[158] It triggers maturation, being responsible for a range of biochemical and cytoarchitectural changes which occur in fetal tissues towards term, in preparation for extrauterine life. It may also signal nutrient insufficiency in the fetus because fetal cortisol levels rise in response to undernutrition. Postnatal glucocorticoid concentrations, at least in the rat, influence the development of the brain.[159]

Interest in the possible long term effects of fetal exposure to glucocorticoids has been stimulated by findings that treatment of pregnant rats with low dose dexamethasone leads to persistently raised blood pressure in the offspring. The mechanisms underlying this are unclear, but may represent the effects of maternal steroids on the mechanisms that control fetal blood pressure.[160] Under normal conditions, glucocorticoids in the maternal circulation are prevented from gaining access to the fetus by a placental enzyme, 11β-hydroxysteroid dehydrogenase, which catalyses the rapid metabolism of cortisol and corticosteroid to inactive products.[161] In rats the activity of this enzyme in the placenta is lowest in neonates who have large placentas but a low birthweight.[160] As described in chapter 4, humans who have a high ratio of placental weight to birthweight have raised blood pressure in adult life.[162]

Thyroid hormones—These hormones have an important role in cell differentiation, and may also be involved in matching fetal oxygen consumption to the oxygen supply. In newborn rats, changes in the serum concentrations of thyroid hormones may permanently change the sensitivity of the hypothalamic–pituitary axis to the hormone.[163-165] In this way the level of negative feedback between the hypothalamus and thyroid gland becomes reset. In the newborn baboon thyroid homoeostasis may likewise be reset by the thyroid hormones in the mother's milk.[127] In adult humans circulating levels of thyroxine and thyroid stimulating hormone (TSH) are related to birthweight and infant feeding. (These findings are described in chapter 5.) This suggests that thyroid function may be set during fetal growth and infant feeding.[166]

Sex hormones—Fifty years ago experiments in rats showed that in early life the hypophysis is plastic and able to differentiate as either male or female, depending on whether or not a testis is present.[167] Low concentrations of androgens during a sensitive perinatal phase imprint the hypothalamus so that gonadotrophin is secreted in cycles, which is the characteristic female pattern; high concentrations of androgens result in continuous "tonic" secretion of gonadotrophin, which is the male pattern.[168] Soon after birth, manipulation of androgen or oestrogen concentrations during sensitive periods changes sexual behaviour of males and females permanently, leading to reduced sexual drive and behaviour that is interpreted as homosexual.[62] In females it also changes sexual physiology, producing anovulatory sterility and polycystic ovaries.[2 169] Remarkably, female rats may be masculinised *in utero* merely by the presence of male littermates sharing the same uterine horn, perhaps because masculinising hormones are carried from the males through the intrauterine vasculature.[170]

IMMUNE SYSTEM

The thymus seems to be particularly sensitive to fetal and neonatal undernutrition. In the rat the size and DNA content of the thymus are permanently reduced by transient undernutrition during pregnancy and early lactation.[3 36 171] Undernutrition also impairs development of thymic derived T lymphocytes and humoral immunity.[172-174] Reduced immune responses in animals can be produced by maternal protein–energy malnutrition[175 176] or deficiency of specific nutrients such as iron and selenium.[171 177] Undernutrition in one generation may affect immunity in the next two generations.[175]

In humans impaired fetal nutrition throughout gestation leads to growth retarded babies who have low birthweight, global impairment of thymic development, and increased susceptibility to infection.[174 178 179] Undernutrition in late gestation may be associated with the diversion of blood and nutrients to the brain at the expense of the trunk.[180] In these babies, who tend to have disproportionately small body size at birth in relation to head size, the weight of the thymus may be severely reduced.[181 182] In the post-term fetus there is a selective and marked wasting of the thymus.[183]

A recent study has shown that middle aged men and women who had disproportionately small body size at birth have persistently raised serum IgE concentrations.[42] It was suggested that this may be linked to an imbalance in thymic derived T lymphocytes.

There is a considerable body of evidence which suggests that the method of infant feeding and the age at weaning influence the later occurrence of allergic disease:[174 184–188] specifically, some studies have shown that breast feeding is associated with reduced occurrence of these diseases.[184 189 190] Studies in pre-term infants have shown that breast milk reduces a range of allergic reactions, including eczema, but only in babies with a family history of atopy.[191]

1 Lucas A. Programming by early nutrition in man. In: Bock GR, Whelan J, eds, *The childhood environment and adult disease*. Chichester: John Wiley & Sons, 1991:38–55.

2 Barraclough CA. Production of anovulatory, sterile rats by single injections of testosterone propionate. *Endocrinology* 1961;**68**:62–7.

3 Winick M, Noble A. Cellular response in rats during malnutrition at various ages. *J Nutr* 1966;**89**:300–6.

4 Roeder LM, Chow BF. Influence of the dietary history of test animals on responses in pharmacological and nutritional studies. *Am J Clin Nutr* 1971;**24**:947–51.

5 Osofsky HJ. Relationships between nutrition during pregnancy and subsequent infant and child development. *Obstet Gynecol Surv* 1975;**30**:227–41.

6 Stephens DN. Growth and the development of dietary obesity in adulthood of rats which have been undernourished during development. *Br J Nutr* 1980;**44**:215–27.

7 Hahn P. Effect of litter size on plasma cholesterol and insulin and some liver and adipose tissue enzymes in adult rodents. *J Nutr* 1984;**114**:1231–4.

8 Swenne I, Crace CJ, Milner RDG. Persistent impairment of insulin secretory response to glucose in adult rats after limited periods of protein-calorie malnutrition early in life. *Diabetes* 1987;**36**:454–8.

9 Hahn P. Late effects of early nutrition. In: Subbiah MTR, ed., *Atherosclerosis: a pediatric perspective*. Florida: CRC Press, 1989:155–64.

10 Mott GE, Lewis DS, McGill HC. Programming of cholesterol metabolism by breast or formula feeding. In: Bock GR, Whelan J, eds, *The childhood environment and adult disease*. Chichester: Wiley, 1991:56–76.

11 Smart JL. Critical periods in brain development. In: Bock GR, Whelan J, eds, *The childhood environment and adult disease*. Chichester: Wiley, 1991:109–28.

12 Widdowson EM, McCance RA. A review: new thoughts on growth. *Pediatr Res* 1975; **9**:154–6.

13 Tanner JM. *Foetus into man: physical growth from conception to maturity*. Ware: Castlemead Publications, 1978.

14 Lorenz K. *King Solomon's ring*. New York: Crowell, 1952.

15 Deeming DC, Ferguson MWJ. Physiological effects of incubation temperature on embryonic development in reptiles and birds. In: Deeming DC, Ferguson MWJ, eds, *Egg incubation: its effects on embryonic development in birds and reptiles*. Cambridge: Cambridge University Press, 1991:147–71.

16 Deeming DC, Ferguson MWJ. The mechanism of temperature dependent sex determination in crocodilians: a hypothesis. *American Zoologist* 1989;**29**:973–85.

17 Widdowson EM. Intra-uterine growth retardation in the pig. 1. Organ size and cellular development at birth and after growth to maturity. *Biol Neonate* 1971;**19**:329–40.

18 Milner RDG. Mechanisms of overgrowth. In: Sharp F, Fraser RB, Milner RDG, eds, *Fetal growth. Proceedings of the 20th study group of the Royal College of Obstetricians and*

Gynaecologists. London: Royal College of Obstetricians and Gynaecologists, 1989: 139–57.

19 Hammond J, Appleton AB. *Growth and the development of mutton qualities in the sheep. A survey of the problems involved in meat production*. Edinburgh: Oliver and Boyd, 1932:112–39.

20 Hellerström C, Swenne I, Andersson A. Islet cell replication and diabetes. In: Lefebvre PJ, Pipeleers DG, eds, *The pathology of the endocrine pancreas in diabetes*. Heidelberg: Springer, 1988:141–70.

21 Hinchliffe SA, Lynch MRJ, Sargent PH, Howard CV, Van Velzen D. The effect of intrauterine growth retardation on the development of renal nephrons. *Br J Obstet Gynaecol* 1992;**99**:296–301.

22 Chow BF, Lee C-J. Effect of dietary restriction of pregnant rats on body weight gain of the offspring. *J Nutr* 1964;**82**:10–18.

23 Dubos R, Savage D, Schaedler R. Biological Freudianism—Lasting effects of early environmental influences. *Pediatrics* 1966;**38**:789–800.

24 Winick M, Noble A. Cellular response with increased feeding in neonatal rats. *J Nutr* 1967;**91**:179–82.

25 Blackwell B-N, Blackwell RQ, Yu TTS, Weng Y-S, Chow BF. Further studies on growth and feed utilization in progeny of underfed mother rats. *J Nutr* 1969;**97**:79–84.

26 Zeman FJ, Stanbrough EC. Effect of maternal protein deficiency on cellular development in the fetal rat. *J Nutr* 1969;**99**:274–82.

27 McLeod KI, Goldrick RB, Whyte HM. The effect of maternal malnutrition on the progeny in the rat. *Aust J Exp Biol Med Sci* 1972;**50**:435–46.

28 Roeder LM. Effect of the level of nutrition on rates of cell proliferation and of RNA and protein syntheses in the rat. *Nutrition Reports International* 1973;7:271–87.

29 Lemonnier D, Suquet J-P, Aubert R, Rosselin G. Long term effect of mouse neonate food intake on adult body composition, insulin and glucose serum levels. *Horm Metab Res* 1973;5:223–4.

30 McCance RA, Widdowson EM. The determinants of growth and form. *Proc R Soc Lond [Biol]* 1974;**185**:1–17.

31 Smart JL, Massey RF, Nash SC, Tonkiss J. Effects of early-life undernutrition in artificially reared rats: subsequent body and organ growth. *Br J Nutr* 1987;**58**:245–55.

32 Widdowson EM, McCance RA. The effect of finite periods of undernutrition at different ages on the composition and subsequent development of the rat. *Proc R Soc Lond [Biol]* 1963;**158**:329–42.

33 McCance RA, Widdowson EM. Nutrition and growth. *Proc R Soc Lond [Biol]* 1962;**156**:326–37.

34 Wigglesworth JS. Experimental growth retardation in the foetal rat. *J Pathol Bacteriol* 1964;**88**:1–13.

35 Roux JM, Tordet-Caridroit C, Chanez C. Studies on experimental hypotrophy in the rat. I. Chemical composition of the total body and some organs in the rat foetus. *Biol Neonate* 1970;**15**:342–7.

36 Moment GB. The effects of rate of growth on the post-natal development of the white rat. *J Exp Zool* 1933;**65**:359–93.

37 Harding J, Liu L, Evans P, Oliver M, Gluckman P. Intrauterine feeding of the growth retarded fetus: can we help? *Early Hum Dev* 1992;**29**:193–7.

38 Clarke MF, Smith AH. Recovery following suppression of growth in the rat. *J Nutr* 1938;**15**:245–56.

39 Brown SA, Rogers LK, Dunn JK, Gotto AM, Patsch W. Development of cholesterol homeostatic memory in the rat is influenced by maternal diets. *Metabolism* 1990;**39**:468–73.

40 Winick M, Fish I, Rosso P. Cellular recovery in rat tissues after a brief period of neonatal malnutrition. *J Nutr* 1968;**95**:623–6.

41 Widdowson EM, Crabb DE, Milner RDG. Cellular development of some human organs before birth. *Arch Dis Child* 1972;**47**:652–5.

42 Godfrey KM, Barker DJP, Osmond C. Disproportionate fetal growth and raised IGE concentrations in adult life. *Clin Exp Allergy* 1994; in press.

43 Snoeck A, Remacle C, Reusens B, Hoet JJ. Effect of a low protein diet during pregnancy on the fetal rat endocrine pancreas. *Biol Neonate* 1990;**57**:107–18.

44 Nagy SU, Csaba G. Dose dependence of the thyrotrophin (TSH) receptor damaging effect of gonadotrophin in the newborn rats. *Acta Physiologica Academiae Scientiarum Hungaricae* 1980;**56**:417–20.

45 Csaba G, Török O. Influence of insulin and biogenic amines on the division of Chang liver cells after primary exposure (imprinting) and repeated treatments. *Cytobios* 1991;**66**:153–6.

46 Csaba G. Phylogeny and ontogeny of hormone receptors: the selection theory of receptor formation and hormonal imprinting. *Biol Rev* 1980;**55**:47–63.

47 Kahn AJ. Embryogenic effect on post-natal changes in hemoglobin concentration with time. *Growth* 1968;**32**:13–22.

48 McCay CM, Maynard LA, Sperling G, Barnes LL. Retarded growth, lifespan, ultimate body size and age changes in the albino rat after feeding diets restricted in calories. *J Nutr* 1939;**18**:1–13.

49 Ross MH. Protein, calories and life expectancy. *Fed Proc* 1959;**18**:1190–207.

50 Berg BN, Simms HS. Nutrition and longevity in the rat. II. Longevity and onset of disease with different levels of food intake. *J Nutr* 1960;**71**:255–63.

51 Comfort A. Nutrition and longevity in animals. *Proc Nutr Soc* 1960;**19**:125–9.

52 Widdowson EM, McCance RA. Some effects of accelerating growth. I. General somatic development. *Proc R Soc Lond [Biol]* 1960;**152**:188–206.

53 Ross MH. Aging, nutrition and hepatic enzyme activity patterns in the rat. *J Nutr* 1969;**97**(suppl 1):563–601.

54 Kirkwood TBL, Cremer T. Cytogerontology since 1881: A reappraisal of August Weismann and a review of modern progress. *Hum Genet* 1982;**60**:101–21.

55 Davis RL, Hargen SM, Yeomans FM, Chow BF. Long term effects of alterations of maternal diet in mice. *Nutrition Reports International* 1973;**7**:463–73.

56 El Habet A, Aust L, Noack R. The influence of postnatal nutrition on lipoprotein lipase activity and hormone sensitive lipolysis in vitro of rat adipose tissue. *Acta Biologica et Medica Germanica* 1979;**38**:601–9.

57 Duff DA, Snell K. Effect of altered neonatal nutrition on the development of enzymes of lipid and carbohydrate metabolism in the rat. *J Nutr* 1982;**112**:1057–66.

58 Lewis DS, Bertrand HA, McMahan CA, McGill HC, Carey KD, Masoro EJ. Preweaning food intake influences the adiposity of young adult baboons. *J Clin Invest* 1986;**78**:899–905.

59 Charney E, Goodman HC, McBride M, Lyon B, Pratt R. Childhood antecedents of adult obesity. *N Engl J Med* 1976;**295**:6–9.

60 Stein ZA, Susser MW. The Dutch Famine 1944–45 and the reproductive process. I. Effects on six indices at birth. *Paediatr Res* 1975;**9**:70–6.

61 Ravelli G-P, Stein ZA, Susser MW. Obesity in young men after famine exposure in utero and early infancy. *N Engl J Med* 1976;**295**:349–53.

62 Dörner G. Environment-dependent brain differentiation and fundamental processes of life. *Acta Biologica et Medica Germanica* 1974;**33**:129–48.

63 Knittle JL, Hirsch J. Effect of early nutrition on the development of rat epididymal fat pads: cellularity and metabolism. *J Clin Invest* 1968;**47**:2091–8.

64 Faust IM, Johnson PR, Stern JS, Hirsch J. Diet-induced adipocyte number increase in adult rats: a new model of obesity. *Am J Physiol* 1978;**235**:E279–86.

65 Winick M, Rosso P, Brasel JA. Malnutrition and cellular growth in the brain: existence of critical periods. In: *Lipids, malnutrition and the developing brain*. New York: Associated Scientific, 1972:199–212.

66 Davies PA, Stewart AL. Low-birthweight infants: neurological sequelae and later intelligence. *Br Med Bull* 1975;**31**:85–91.

67 Katz HB. The influence of undernutrition on learning performance in rodents. *Nutrition Abstracts and Reviews Series 'A'* 1980;**50**:767–84.

68 Patel AJ, Balazs R, Smith RM, Kingsbury AE, Hunt A. Thyroid hormone and brain development. In: Di Benedetta C, ed., *Multidisciplinary approach to brain development*. Amsterdam: Elsevier, 1980:261–77.

69 Davison AN, Dobbing J. Myelination as a vulnerable period in brain development. *Br Med Bull* 1966;**22**:40–4.

70 Smart JL. Early life malnutrition and later learning ability. A critical analysis. In: Oliverio A, ed. *Genetics, environment and intelligence*. Amsterdam: Elsevier, 1977:215–35.

71 Boothe RG, Dobson V, Teller DY. Postnatal development of vision in human and nonhuman primates. *Annu Rev Neurosci* 1985;**8**:495–545.

72 Blakemore C. Sensitive and vulnerable periods in the development of the visual system. In: Bock GR, Whelan J, eds. *The childhood environment and adult disease*. Chichester: Wiley, 1991:129–54.

73 Lucas A, Morley R, Cole TJ, Gore SM, Lucas PJ, Crowle P, Pearse R, Boon AJ, Powell R. Early diet in preterm babies and developmental status at 18 months. *Lancet* 1990;**335**:1477–81.

74 Lucas A. Influence of neonatal nutrition on long-term outcome. In: Salle BL, Swyer PR, eds. *Nestlé Nutrition Workshop Series*, Vol. 32. New York: Raven Press, 1993:181–96.

75 Goswami T, Vu M-L, Srivastava U. Quantitative changes in DNA, RNA and protein content of the various organs of the young of undernourished female rats. *J Nutr* 1974;**104**:1257–64.

76 Bassi JA, Rosso P, Moessinger AC, Blanc WA, James LS. Fetal growth retardation due to maternal tobacco smoke exposure in the rat. *Pediatr Res* 1984;**18**:127–30.

77 Collins MH, Moessinger AC, Kleinerman J *et al*. Fetal lung hypoplasia associated with maternal smoking: a morphometric analysis. *Pediatr Res* 1985;**19**:408–12.

78 Lechner AJ, Winston DC, Bauman JE. Lung mechanics, cellularity and surfactant after prenatal starvation in guinea pigs. *J Appl Physiol* 1986;**60**:1610–14.

79 Faridy EE, Sanii MR, Thliveris JA. Fetal lung growth: influence of maternal hypoxia and hyperoxia in rats. *Respir Physiol* 1988;**73**:225–41.

80 O'Dell BL, Kilburn KH, McKenzie WN, Thurston RJ. The lung of the copper-deficient rat. *Am J Pathol* 1978;**91**:413–32.

81 Das RM. The effects of intermittent starvation on lung development in suckling rats. *Am J Pathol* 1984;**117**:326–32.

82 Sahebjami H, MacGee J. Effects of starvation on lung mechanics and biochemistry in young and old rats. *J Appl Physiol* 1985;**58**:778–84.

83 Kalenga M, Eeckhout Y. Effects of protein deprivation from the neonatal period on lung collagen and elastin in the rat. *Pediatr Res* 1989;**26**:125–7.

84 Matsui R, Thurlbeck WM, Fujita Y, Yu SY, Kida K. Connective tissue, mechanical, and morphometric changes in the lungs of weanling rats fed a low protein diet. *Pediatric Pulmonology* 1989;**7**:159–66.

85 Lechner AJ, Banchero N. Advanced pulmonary development in newborn guinea pigs (*Cavia porcellus*). *Am J Anat* 1982;**163**:235–46.

86 Lechner AJ. Perinatal age determines the severity of retarded lung development induced by starvation. *Am Rev Respir Dis* 1985;**131**:638–43.

87 Gaultier C. Malnutrition and lung growth. *Pediatric Pulmonology* 1991;**10**:278–86.

88 Winick M, Noble A. Quantitative changes in DNA, RNA and protein during prenatal and postnatal growth in the rat. *Dev Biol* 1965;**12**:451–6.

89 Burri P, Dbaly J, Weibel ER. The postnatal growth of the rat lung. I. Morphometry. *Anat Rec* 1974;**178**:711–30.

90 Bucher U, Reid L. Development of the intrasegmental tree; the pattern of branching and development of cartilage at various stages of intrauterine life. *Thorax* 1961;**16**:207–18.

91 Wigglesworth JS, Desai R. Is fetal respiratory function a major determinant of perinatal survival? *Lancet* 1982;**i**:264–7.

92 Kitterman JA. Fetal lung development. *J Dev Physiol* 1984;**6**:67–82.

93 Moessinger AC, Bassi GA, Ballantyne G, Collins MH, James LS, Blanc WA. Experimental production of pulmonary hypoplasia following amniocentesis and oligohydramnios. *Early Hum Dev* 1983;**8**:343–50.

94 Nakayama DK, Glick PL, Harrison MR, Villa RL, Noall R. Experimental pulmonary hypoplasia due to oligohydramnios and its reversal by relieving thoracic compression. *J Pediatr Surg* 1983;**18**:347–53.

95 Higuchi M, Kato T, Matsuda K, *et al.* The influence of experimentally produced oligohydramnios on lung growth and pulmonary surfactant content in fetal rabbits. *J Dev Physiol* 1991;**16**:223–7.

96 Moessinger AC, Harding R, Adamson TM, Singh M, Kiu GT. Role of lung liquid fluid volume in growth and maturation of the fetal sheep lung. *J Clin Invest* 1990;**86**:1270–77.

97 Fisk NM, Parkes MJ, Moore PJ, Haidar A, Wigglesworth J, Hanson MA. Fetal breathing during chronic lung liquid loss leading to pulmonary hypoplasia. *Early Hum Dev* 1991;**27**:53–63.

98 Wigglesworth JS, Desai R, Guerrini P. Fetal lung hypoplasia: biochemical and structural variations and their possible significance. *Arch Dis Child* 1981;**56**:606–15.

99 Nimrod C, Varela-Gittings F, Machin G, Campbell D, Wesenberg R. The effect of very prolonged membrane rupture on fetal development. *Am J Obstet Gynecol* 1984;**148**:540–3.

100 Roberts AB, Mitchell JM. Direct ultrasonographic measurements of fetal lung length in normal pregnancies and pregnancies complicated by prolonged rupture of membranes. *Am J Clin Nutr* 1990;**163**:1560–6.

101 Hislop A, Reid L. Persistent hypoplasia of the lung after repair of congenital diaphragmatic hernia. *Thorax* 1976;**31**:452–5.

102 Helms P, Stocks J. Lung function in infants with congenital pulmonary hypoplasia. *J Pediatr* 1982;**101**:918–22.

103 Thurlbeck WM. Prematurity and the developing lung. *Clinical Perinatology* 1992;**19**:497–519.

104 Davies G, Reid L. Effect of scoliosis on growth of alveoli and pulmonary arteries and on right ventricle. *Arch Dis Child* 1971;**46**:623–32.

105 Owage-Iraka JW, Harrison A, Warner JO. Lung function in congenital and idiopathic scoliosis. *Eur J Pediatr* 1984;**142**:198–200.

106 Zeman FJ. Effects of maternal protein restriction on the kidney of the newborn young of rats. *J Nutr* 1968;**94**:111–16.

107 Langley SC, Jackson AA. Increased systolic blood pressure in adult rats induced by fetal exposure to maternal low protein diets. *Clin Sci* 1994;**86**:217–22.

108 Osathanondh V, Potter EL. Development of human kidney as shown by microdissection. III. Formation and interrelationships of collecting tubules and nephrons. *Arch Pathol* 1963;**76**:290–302.

109 Shrader RE, Zeman FJ. Effect of maternal protein deprivation on morphological and enzymatic development of neonatal rat tissue. *J Nutr* 1969;**99**:401–21.

110 Innis SM. The role of diet during development on the regulation of adult cholesterol homeostasis. *Can J Physiol Pharmacol* 1985;**63**:557–64.

111 Reiser R, Sidelman Z. Control of serum homeostasis by cholesterol in the milk of the suckling rat. *J Nutr* 1972;**102**:1009–16.

112 Reiser R, Henderson GR, O'Brien BC. Persistence of dietary suppression of 3-hydroxy-3-methylglutaryl coenzyme-A reductase during development in rats. *J Nutr* 1977;**107**:1131–8.

113 Kris-Etherton PM, Layman DK, York PV, Frantz ID. The influence of early nutrition on the serum cholesterol of the adult rat. *J Nutr* 1979;**109**:1244–57.

114 Li JR, Bale LK, Kottke BA. Effect of neonatal modulation of cholesterol homeostasis on subsequent response to cholesterol challenge in adult guinea pig. *J Clin Invest* 1980;**65**:1060–8.

115 Green MH, Dohner EL, Green JB. Influence of dietary fat and cholesterol on milk lipids and on cholesterol metabolism in the rat. *J Nutr* 1981;**111**:276–86.

116 Innis SM. Influence of maternal cholestyramine treatment on cholesterol and bile metabolism in adult offspring. *J Nutr* 1983;**113**:2464–70.

117 Little M-T, Hahn P. Diet and metabolic development. *FASEB J* 1990;**4**:2605–11.

118 Hassan AS, Yunker RL, Subbiah MTR. Decreased bile acid pool in neonates of guinea pigs fed cholesterol during pregnancy. *J Nutr* 1981;**111**:2030–3.

119 Hassan AS, Gallon LS, Yunker BS, Subbiah MTR. Effect of enhancement of cholesterol catabolism in guinea pigs after weaning on subsequent response to dietary cholesterol. *Am J Clin Nutr* 1982;**35**:546–50.

120 O'Brien BC, McMurray DN, Reiser R. The influence of premature weaning and the nature of the fat in the diet during development on adult plasma lipids and adipose cellularity in pair-fed rats. *J Nutr* 1983;**113**:602–9.

121 Angel JF, Back DW. Weaning and metabolic regulation in the rat. *Can J Physiol Pharmacol* 1985;**63**:538–45.

122 Hahn P. Obesity and atherosclerosis as consequences of early weaning. In: Ballabriga A, Rey J, eds, *Weaning: Why, what, and when?* New York: Vevey/Raven Press, 1987: 93–109.

123 Hahn, P, Kirby L. Immediate and late effects of premature weaning and of feeding a high fat or high carbohydrate diet to weanling rats. *J Nutr* 1973;**103**:690–6.

124 Villalon L, Tuchweber B, Yousef IM. Low protein diets potentiate lithocholic acid-induced cholestasis in rats. *J Nutr* 1992;**122**:1587–96.

125 Mott GE, Jackson EM, McMahan CA, McGill HC. Cholesterol metabolism in adult baboons is influenced by infant diet. *J Nutr* 1990;**120**:243–51.

126 Mott GE, Lewis DS, McGill HC. Deferred effects of preweaning nutrition on lipid metabolism. *Ann NY Acad Sci* 1991;**6**:70–80.

127 Lewis DS, McMahan CA, Mott GE. Breast feeding and formula feeding affect differently plasma thyroid hormone concentrations in infant baboons. *Biol Neonate* 1993;**63**:327–35.

128 Hahn Jr, H. B., Spiekermen AM, Otto WR, Hossalla DE. Thyroid function tests in neonates fed human milk. *Am J Dis Child* 1983;**137**:220–2.

129 Franklin R, O'Grady C, Carpenter L. Neonatal thyroid function: comparison between breast-fed and bottle-fed infants. *J Pediatr* 1985;**106**:124–6.

130 Oberkotter LV, Periera GR, Paul MH, Ling H, Sasahow S, Farber M. Effect of breast-feeding vs formula-feeding on circulating thyroxine levels in premature infants. *J Pediatr* 1985;**106**:822–5.

131 Fomon SJ, Bartels DJ. Concentrations of cholesterol in serum of infants in relation to diet. *AMA J Dis Child* 1960;**99**:27–30.

132 Darmady JM, Fosbrooke AS, Lloyd JK. Prospective study of serum cholesterol levels during first year of life. *BMJ* 1972;**2**:685–8.

133 Andersen GE, Lifschitz C, Friis-Hansen B. Dietary habits and serum lipids during first 4 years of life. *Acta Paediatr Scand* 1979;**68**:165–70.

134 Van Biervliet JP, Rosseneu M, Caster H. Influence of dietary factors on the plasma lipoprotein composition and content in neonates. *Eur J Pediatr* 1986;**144**:489–93.

135 Labarthe DR, Eissa M, Vara C. Childhood precursors of high blood pressure and elevated cholesterol. *Annu Rev Public Health* 1991;**12**:519–41.

136 Sporik R, Johnstone JH, Cogswell JJ. Longitudinal study of cholesterol values in 68 children from birth to 11 years of age. *Arch Dis Child* 1991;**66**:134–7.

137 Fall CHD, Barker DJP, Osmond C, Winter PD, Clark PMS, Hales CN. Relation of infant feeding to adult serum cholesterol concentration and death from ischaemic heart disease. *BMJ* 1992;**304**:801–5.

138 Barker DJP, Martyn CN, Osmond C, Hales CN, Fall CHD. Growth in utero and serum cholesterol concentrations in adult life. *BMJ* 1993;**307**:1524–7.

139 Chow BF, Blackwell RQ, Blackwell B, Hou TY, Anilane JK, Sherwin RW. Maternal nutrition and metabolism of the offspring: studies in rats and man. *Am J Public Health* 1968;**58**:668–77.

140 Hsueh AM, Blackwell RQ, Chow BF. Effect of maternal diet in rats on feed consumption in the offspring. *J Nutr* 1970;**100**:1157–64.

141 Fowden AL. The role of insulin in prenatal growth. *J Dev Physiol* 1989;**12**:173–82.

142 Fowden AL. Pancreatic endocrinology, function and carbohydrate metabolism in the fetus. In: Albrecht E, Pepe GJ eds, *Perinatal endocrinology*, Vol. IV, *Research in perinatal medicine*. 1985:71–90.

143 Heard CRC, Henry PAJ. The insulinogenic response to intravenous glucose in dogs fed diets of different protein value. *J Endocrinol* 1969;**45**:375–86.

144 Turner MR. Protein deficiency, reproduction, and hormonal factors in growth. *Nutrition Reports International* 1973;**7**:289–95.

145 van Assche FA, Aerts L. Long-term effects of diabetes and pregnancy in the rat. *Diabetes* 1985;**34**(suppl 2):116–18.

146 Aerts L, Holemans K, van Assche FA. Maternal diabetes during pregnancy: consequences for the offspring. *Diabetes/Metabolism Reviews* 1990;**6**:147–67.

147 van Assche FA, Aerts L. The fetal endocrine pancreas. *Contrib Gynecol Obstet* 1979;**5**: 44–57.

148 Gluckman PD, Gunn AJ, Wray A, *et al.* Congenital idiopathic growth hormone deficiency is associated with prenatal and early postnatal growth failure. *J Pediatr* 1992;**121**:920–3.

149 Stephan JK, Chow B, Frohman LA, Chow BF. Relationship of growth hormone to the growth retardation associated with maternal dietary restriction. *J Nutr* 1971;**101**: 1453–8.

150 Zeman FJ, Shrader RE, Allen LH. Persistent effects of maternal protein deficiency in postnatal rats. *Nutrition Reports International* 1973;**7**:421–36.

151 Bassett NS, Oliver MH, Breier BH, Gluckman PD. The effect of maternal starvation on plasma insulin-like growth factor 1 concentrations in the late gestation ovine fetus. *Pediatr Res* 1990;**27**:401–4.

152 Oliver MH, Harding JE, Breier BH, Evans PC, Gluckman PD. Glucose but not a mixed amino acid infusion regulates plasma insulin-like growth factor-1 concentrations in fetal sheep. *Pediatr Res* 1993;**34**:62–5.

153 Owens JA. Endocrine and substrate control of fetal growth: placental and maternal influences and insulin-like growth factors. *Reproduction Fertility and Development* 1991;**3**:501–7.

154 Furuhashi N, Fukaya T, Kono H, *et al.* Cord serum growth hormone in the human fetus. Sex difference and a negative correlation with birth weight. *Gynecol Obstet Invest* 1983;**16**:119–24.

155 Thieriot-Prevost G, Boccara JF, Francoual C, Badoual J, Job JC. Serum insulin-like growth factor 1 and serum growth-promoting activity during the first postnatal year in infants with intrauterine growth retardation. *Pediatr Res* 1988;**24**:380–3.

156 Deiber M, Chatelain P, Naville D, Putet G, Salle B. Functional hypersomatotropism in small for gestational age (SGA) newborn infants. *J Clin Endocrinol Metab* 1989;**68**: 232–4.

157 Law CM, Barker DJP, Hales CN, Shiell AW, Normand ICS. Insulin resistance in 7 year old children who were thin at birth. *Pediatr Res* 1994;**35**:263.

158 Silver M. Prenatal maturation, the timing of birth and how it may be regulated in domestic animals. *Experimental Physiology* 1990;**75**:285–307.

159 Sapolski RM, Meaney MJ. Maturation of the adrenocortical stress response: neuroendocrine control mechanisms and the stress hyporesponsive period. *Brain Res Rev* 1986;**11**:65–76.

160. Benediktsson R, Lindsay RS, Noble J, Seckl JR, Edwards CRW. Glucocorticoid exposure in utero: new model for adult hypertension. *Lancet* 1993;**341**:339–41.

161 Edwards CRW, Benediktsson R, Lindsay RS, Seckl JR. Dysfunction of placental glucocorticoid barrier: link between fetal environment and adult hypertension? *Lancet* 1993;**341**:355–7.

162 Barker DJP, Bull AR, Osmond C, Simmonds SJ. Fetal and placental size and risk of hypertension in adult life. *BMJ* 1990;**301**:259–62.

163 Besa ME, Pascual-Leone AM. Effect of neonatal hyperthyroidism upon the regulation of TSH secretion in rats. *Acta Endocrinol* 1984;**105**:31–9.

164 Walker P, Courtin F. Transient neonatal hyperthyroidism results in hypothyroidism in the adult rat. *Endocrinology* 1985;**116**:2246–50.

165 Pracyk JB, Seidler FJ, McCook EC, Slotkin TA. Pituitary-thyroid axis reactivity to hyper- and hypothyroidism in the perinatal period: ontogeny of regulation and long-term programming of responses. *J Dev Physiol* 1992;**18**:105–9.

166 Phillips DIW, Barker DJP, Osmond C. Infant feeding, fetal growth and adult thyroid function. *Acta Endocrinol* 1993;**129**:134–6.

167 Pfeiffer CA. Sexual differences of the hypophyses and their determination by the gonads. *Am J Anat* 1936;**58**:195–225.

168 Barraclough CA, Gorski RA. Evidence that the hypothalamus is responsible for androgen-induced sterility in the female rat. *Endocrinology* 1961;**68**:68–79.

169 vom Saal FS, Bronson FH. Sexual characteristics of adult female mice are correlated with their blood testosterone levels during prenatal development. *Science* 1980;**208**: 597–9.

170 Meisel RL, Ward IL. Fetal female rats are masculinized by male littermates located caudally in the uterus. *Science* 1981;**213**:239–42.

171 Kochanowski BA, Sherman AR. Decreased antibody formation in iron-deficient rat pups—effect of iron repletion. *Am J Clin Nutr* 1985;**41**:278–84.

172 Jarrett E, Hall E. Selective suppression of IgE antibody responsiveness by maternal influence. *Nature* 1979;**280**:145–6.

173 Kochanowski BA, Sherman AR. Cellular growth in iron-deficient rats: effect of pre- and post-weaning iron repletion. *J Nutr* 1985;**115**:279–87.

174 Chandra RK. Interactions between early nutrition and the immune system. In: Bock GR, Whelan J, eds, *The childhood environment and adult disease*. Chichester: Wiley, 1991:77–92.

175 Chandra RK. Antibody formation in first and second generation offspring of nutritionally deprived rats. *Science* 1975;**190**:289–90.

176 Srivasta US, Thakur ML, Majumdar PK, Bhatnagar GM, Supakar PC. Lymphoid organ mRNA translatability in rats: effect of protein energy undernutrition in early life. *J Nutr* 1987;**117**:242–6.

177 Mulhearn SA, Taylor GL, Magruder LE, Vessey AR. Deficient levels of dietary selenium suppress the antibody response in first and second generation mice. *Nutrition Research* 1985;**5**:201–10.

178 Chandra RK. Fetal malnutrition and postnatal immunocompetence. *Am J Dis Child* 1975;**129**:450–5.

179 Moscatelli P, Dagna Bricarelli F, Piccinini A, Tomatis C, Dufour MA. Defective immunocompetence in foetal undernutrition. *Helv paediatr Acta* 1976;**31**:241–7.

180 Rudolph AM. The fetal circulation and its response to stress. *J Dev Physiol* 1984;**6**: 11–19.

181 Pauerstein CJ. *Clinical obstetrics*. Edinburgh: Churchill Livingstone, 1987.

182 Owens JA, Owens P, Robinson J. Experimental fetal growth retardation: metabolic and endocrine aspects. In: Gluckman PD, Johnston BM, Nathanielsz PW, eds, *Advances in fetal physiology*. Ithaca, NY: Perinatology Press, 1989:263–86.

183 Gruenwald P. Pathology of the deprived fetus and its supply line. In: Elliott K, Knight J, eds, *Size at birth. Ciba Foundation Symposium No. 27*. Amsterdam: Elsevier, 1975:3–19.

184 Kramer MS, Moroz B. Do breast-feeding and delayed introduction of solid foods protect against subsequent atopic eczema? *J Pediatr* 1981;**98**:546–50.

185 Miskelly FG, Burr ML, Vaughan-Williams E, Fehily AM, Butland BK, Merrett TG. Infant feeding and allergy. *Arch Dis Child* 1988;**63**:388–93.

186 Chandra RK. Long-term health implications of mode of infant feeding. *Nutrition Research* 1989;**9**:1–4.

187 Chandra RK, Singh GK, Shridhara B. Effect of feeding whey hydrolysate, soy and conventional cow milk formulas on incidence of atopic disease in high risk infants. *Ann Allergy* 1989;**63**:102–6.

188 Chandra RK. Long-term health consequences of early infant feeding. In: Atkinson SA, Hanson LA, Chandra RK, eds, *Breastfeeding, nutrition, infection and infant growth in developed and emerging countries*. St Johns, Newfoundland: ARTS Biomedical Publishers, 1990:47–55.

189 Chandra RK, Puri S, Cheema PS. Predictive value of cord blood IgE in the development of atopic disease and role of breast-feeding in its prevention. *Clin Allergy* 1985;**15**:517–22.

190 Kramer MS. Does breast feeding help protect against atopic disease? Biology, methodology, and a golden jubilee of controversy. *J Pediatr* 1988;**112**:181–90.

191 Lucas A, Brooke OG, Morley R, Cole TJ, Bamford MT. Early diet of preterm infants and development of allergic or atopic disease: randomised prospective study. *BMJ* 1990;**300**:837–40.

3: From birth to death

Margaret Burnside's ledgers

To examine the hypothesis that coronary heart disease and stroke are "programmed" *in utero* has required new kinds of epidemiological studies. Evidence from studies of geography and time trends can only be suggestive. To advance the hypothesis by epidemiological methods it is necessary to relate the early growth of individual men and women directly to the later occurrence of cardiovascular disease. This requires studies of people now in middle and late life whose early growth was recorded.

Staff from the Medical Research Council (MRC) searched archives and hospital record departments throughout Britain, looking for maternity and infant welfare records from the early years of the century. Many were found. Some were in large collections preserved over many years; in some there were no more than a few hundred records kept by one clinic or even one midwife. Some were detailed and some perfunctory. Some were in archives; others were in lofts, sheds, garages, boiler rooms, or flooded basements. The largest set of records were those made by health visitors in the county of Hertfordshire from 1911 onwards.

In Britain, in the early years of the century, there was widespread concern about the apparent physical deterioration of the British people. The birth rate was declining. One in ten babies died before they were a year old and many of those who survived reached adult life in poor health. During 1902, reports in the national press claimed that up to two thirds of the young men who volunteered to fight in the South African war had been rejected because of unsatisfactory physique.[1] An interdepartmental committee set up in 1903 drew a shocking picture of the nation's children—malnourished, poorly housed, deprived. The Medical Officer of Health for Hertfordshire, writing at around this time, stated:

> Hertfordshire does less than forty out of the fifty-five counties to perpetuate the national stock; for England and Wales the birth-rate has for thirty-three years been steadily declining, only two Continental countries (Belgium and France) having lower birth-rates in 1909, while that for Japan is increasing and is now ahead of every white race but Russia and three of the Balkan States. The new census figures show a lower rate of increase than in any decennium of the last century. This decay must betoken the doom of modern civilisation as it did that of Rome and Greece, unless some new moral or physical factor arise to defeat it. [He added] it is of national importance that the life of every infant be vigorously conserved.

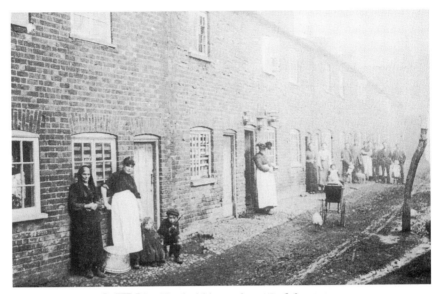

FIG 3.1—*Mothers in Hitchin, Hertfordshire at the turn of the century.*

Miss Ethel Margaret Burnside, the county's first ever "Chief Health Visitor and Lady Inspector of Midwives" set up an "army" of trained nurses to attend women in childbirth and to advise mothers on how to keep their babies healthy. From 1911 onwards when women in Hertfordshire, like those shown in fig 3.1, had their babies, they were attended by a midwife. She recorded the birthweight and notified the birth to the county medical officer of health. The local health visitor was informed. She went to the baby's home at intervals throughout infancy and recorded its illnesses and development on a card. When the baby was one year old the visits ceased; the card was handed in to the county health visitor and the details carefully transferred into ledgers. Fig 3.2 shows a page from one of the ledgers, with birthweight, weight at one year, whether the baby was weaned at one year, number of teeth, and other details. From 1923 onwards the health visitors continued their visits until the child was five years old. Records of these visits were also entered in the ledgers.

The ledgers were maintained until 1945, many years after Miss Burnside had retired. In 1986, the MRC found that those which covered the eastern part of the county had been sent to the County Record Office. Over the next two years those for other areas of the county came to light, preserved in local hospitals.

Surprisingly little is known about Margaret Burnside (1877–1953), whose foresight and dedication have given us the Hertfordshire records. The only known photograph of her (fig 3.3) was taken when she was 17 years old.

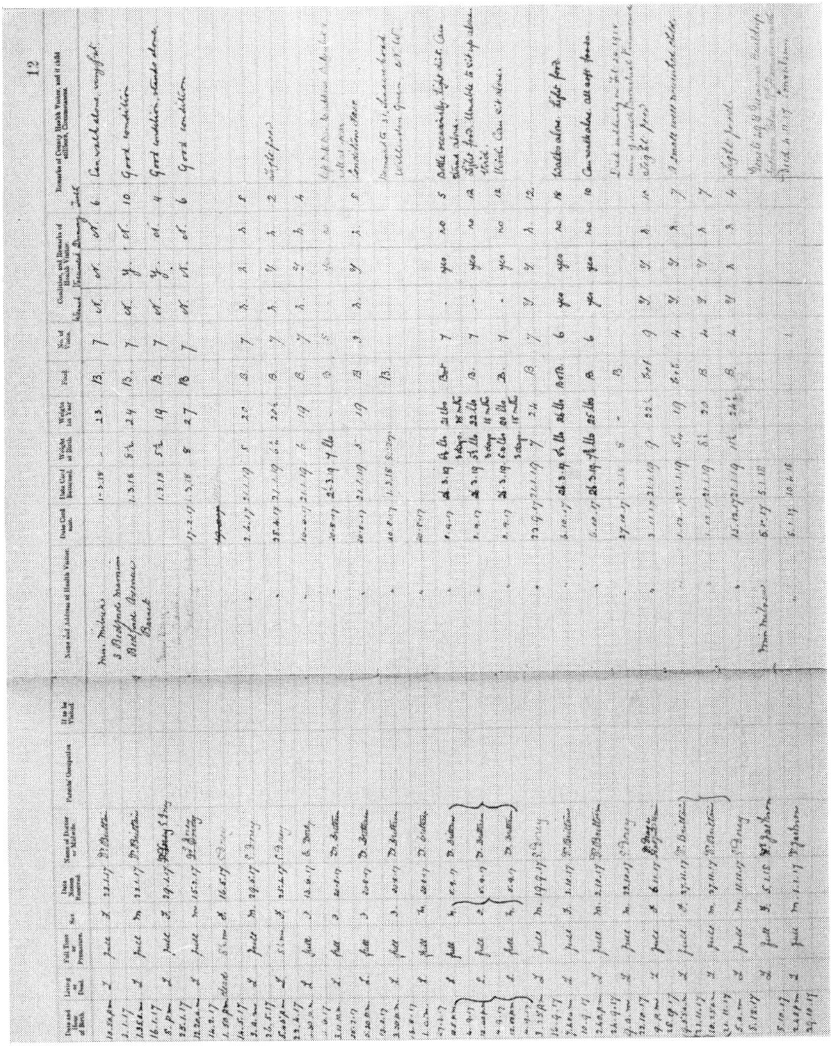

FIG 3.2—*One of Miss Burnside's ledgers in 1917.*

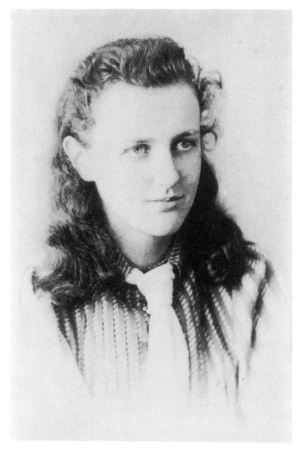

FIG 3.3—*Ethel Margaret Burnside aged 17 years.*

She was born in 1877, one of six children. Her father was rector of Hertingfordbury, a village near Hertford. After training as a nurse at St George's Hospital, London, she became Lady Inspector of Midwives for Hertfordshire in 1905. We know that she worked energetically; "The cyclometer of my bicycle registered 2,921 miles for the year [1907]", she reported. In 1910 she was made a Queen's Nurse and the county nursing association recorded its "high appreciation" of her "unremitting labours". The following year she was appointed as County Health Visitor, following the Notification of Births Act in 1907 which required such an appointment. In 1913 she persuaded the County Council to buy her a car. It was 9·5 horsepower and she called it "little hero".

She is remembered as a reserved but formidable woman. The Clerk to the County Council would make himself immediately available if he knew Miss Burnside was in the building and wished to see him. In 1919 she moved to London, to the newly formed Ministry of Health. Systematic observations of the growth and health of each baby born in Hertfordshire continued for another 25 years.

Early growth and death from cardiovascular disease

The Hertfordshire records made it possible to relate people's early growth, feeding, and illness to their health in later life. The National Health Service Central Register at Southport was used to trace 16 000 men and women born in the county from 1911 to 1930. Tracing required both the forename and surname, and where forenames of the Hertfordshire babies were not recorded they were found through the national index of births or local baptismal registers. In Britain women are more difficult to trace than men because of their change of name at marriage, and it proved impossible to trace most women born before 1923, many of whom married before the Central Register was established in 1939. The study was therefore based on 10 141 men born during 1911–30 and a younger cohort of 5585 women born during 1923–30;[23] 2472 of the men and 690 of the women had died at ages from 20 to 74 years. Of the deaths those of 1172 men and 183 women were the result of cardiovascular disease; 73% of these deaths in

TABLE 3.1—*Standardised mortality ratios among men according to birthweight and weight at one year*

		Cause of death								
		Coronary heart disease		All cardio-vascular disease		All other causes		Lung cancer		All causes	
Weight (lb)*		SMR	*n*	SMR	*n*	SMR	*n*	SMR	*n*	SMR	*n*
Birthweight											
≤5·5	(*n* = 458)	102	51	96	65	90	67	116	19	93	132
−6·5	(*n* = 1317)	83	118	80	155	76	162	64	30	78	317
−7·5	(*n* = 2991)	82	266	80	353	79	383	75	80	80	736
−8·5	(*n* = 3166)	75	266	79	377	77	401	79	92	78	778
−9·5	(*n* = 1505)	56	97	61	144	74	190	57	33	68	334
>9·5	(*n* = 704)	66	55	69	78	79	97	94	26	74	175
One year old											
≤18	(*n* = 559)	105	68	101	89	77	74	98	21	89	163
−20	(*n* = 1702)	83	158	84	217	92	261	89	56	88	478
−22	(*n* = 3288)	85	305	86	420	78	415	73	86	82	835
−24	(*n* = 2754)	65	201	66	277	68	309	58	59	67	586
−26	(*n* = 1359)	65	98	66	135	79	178	92	46	73	313
>26	(*n* = 479)	42	23	46	34	77	63	66	12	62	97
Total	(*n* = 10 141)	76	853	77	1172	78	1300	75	280	77	2472

*1 lb = 454 g.

TABLE 3.2—*Standardised mortality ratios among women according to birthweight and weight at one year*

	Cause of death								
	Coronary heart disease		All cardio-vascular disease		All other causes		Lung cancer		All causes	
Weight (lb)*	SMR	n	SMR	n	SMR	n	SMR	n	SMR	n
Birthweight										
≤5·5	(n= 307)	83	6	80	11	120	38	92	3	108	49
−6·5	(n=1068)	72	19	82	41	72	83	67	8	75	124
−7·5	(n=1956)	67	32	76	69	85	179	88	19	83	248
−8·5	(n=1532)	59	23	63	46	84	141	58	10	78	187
−9·5	(n= 551)	43	6	46	12	87	52	112	7	74	64
>9·5	(n= 171)	49	2	51	4	78	14	0	0	70	18
One year old										
≤18	(n= 617)	91	14	72	21	107	71	87	6	96	92
−20	(n=1486)	54	20	70	49	80	128	78	13	77	177
−22	(n=1926)	68	32	69	61	75	153	75	16	73	214
−24	(n=1103)	47	13	66	34	91	108	57	7	83	142
−26	(n= 353)	76	7	70	12	93	36	99	4	85	48
>26	(n= 100)	76	2	122	6	100	11	87	1	107	17
Total	(n=5585)	63	88	70	183	84	507	76	47	80	690

*1lb=454 g.

men and 48% in women were caused by coronary heart disease. As Hertfordshire is in the south of England, the death rates from cardiovascular disease were below the national average, the standardised mortality ratios being 77 for men and 70 for women.

Tables 3.1 and 3.2 show that, in men and women, standardised mortality rates for cardiovascular disease fell with increasing birthweight. The trends were statistically significant. In men, but not women, there were also strong and highly statistically significant correlations with weight at one year of age. Trends in coronary heart disease were similar to those for all cardiovascular disease, but there were insufficient numbers to allow separate analysis of deaths from stroke. In both men and women there were no trends in non-cardiovascular causes of death or lung cancer (an indicator of cigarette smoking) with birthweight or weight at one year.

Figs 3.4 and 3.5 show the trends in premature death from cardiovascular disease, that is, death under the age of 65 years. Death rates fell progressively from those with birthweight of 5·5 lb or less (≤2·5 kg) to those with birthweight of 9·5 lb (4·3 kg) but increased slightly in those with birthweight more than 9·5 lb (see fig 3.5). The trends with weight at one year of age were different in the two sexes, the large progressive fall among men contrasting with the absence of any trend in women.

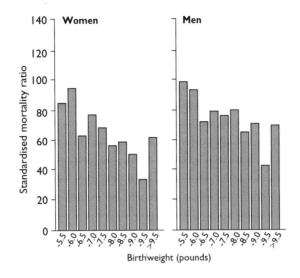

FIG 3.4—*Standardised mortality ratios for cardiovascular disease below the age of 65.*

Table 3.3 shows the simultaneous effects of birthweight and weight at one year of age on premature death from cardiovascular disease. Among women the highest death rates were in those who had below average birthweight, but above average weight at one year of age—that is, their growth "caught up" during infancy. Among men the highest rates were in those who had below average birthweight and below average weight at one year of age—that is, their growth failed to catch up during infancy. Studies of men and women who still live in Hertfordshire have shown that failure of infant weight gain, with a low weight at one year of age, is followed by persisting deficits in growth. Weight at one year of age is closely correlated to adult height, but it is only weakly linked to adult body mass—an index of obesity. The following section suggests how the different associations between cardiovascular disease and pattern of infant growth in women and men can be linked to different body proportions at birth.

The combined effects of birthweight and weight at one year of age on death rates from coronary heart disease in men are shown in fig 3.6; this was derived using Cox's proportional hazards method.[4] The lines join points that have an equal risk of coronary heart disease, and the values are the risks relative to the value of 100 for those with average birthweight and weight at one year of age. Clearly the combination of poor prenatal and

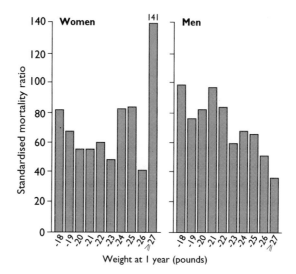

FIG 3.5—*Standardised mortality ratios for cardiovascular disease below the age of 65.*

postnatal growth leads to the highest death rates from coronary heart disease. Birthweight and weight at one year of age are related, although not as strongly as is sometimes suggested (the correlation coefficient was

TABLE 3.3—*Standardised mortality ratios for cardiovascular disease below 65 years according to birthweight and weight at one year*

Birthweight (lb)*	Weight at one year (lb)			
	≤21	22–23	≥24	All
Men				
≤7	97 (170)	81 (76)	62 (39)	86 (285)
7·5–8·5	89 (138)	71 (122)	63 (90)	75 (350)
≥9	73 (36)	73 (53)	57 (62)	66 (151)
All	90 (344)	74 (251)	61 (191)	76 (786)
Women				
≤7	68 (41)	81 (16)	88 (7)	73 (64)
7·5–8·5	63 (30)	51 (15)	78 (12)	62 (57)
≥9	36 (3)	20 (2)	92 (8)	48 (13)
All	63 (74)	56 (33)	84 (27)	65 (134)

*1 lb = 454 g.
Figures in parentheses are numbers of deaths.

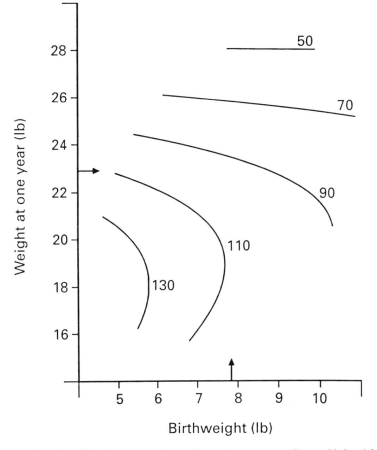

FIG 3.6—*Relative risks for coronary heart disease in men according to birthweight and weight at one year. Lines join points with equal risk. Arrows = mean weights.*

0·36 in Hertfordshire). Few men with low birthweight attained the heavier weights at one year of age, and hence the lowest risks of coronary heart disease.

Body proportions at birth and death from cardiovascular disease

The Hertfordshire records did not include measurements of body size at birth, other than weight, nor did they include length of gestation. Body proportions at birth, for example, weight in relation to length, are important because they indicate the time in gestation at which growth was restrained. Chapter 2 described studies of animals which have shown that, although

45

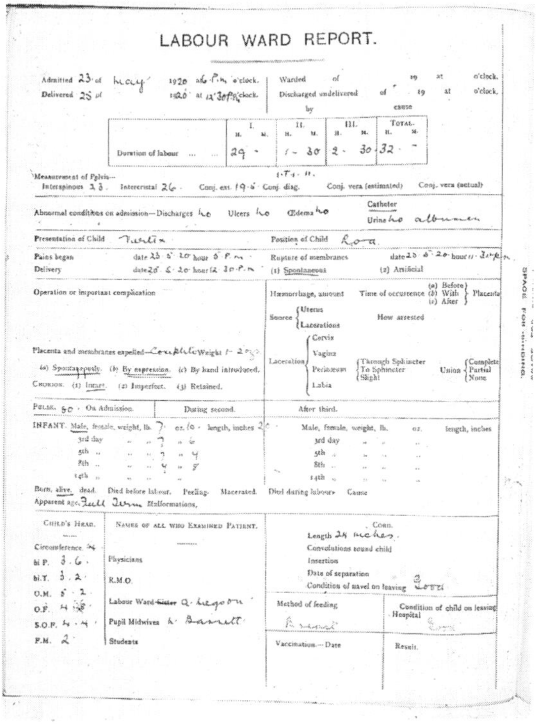

LABOUR WARD REPORT.

Admitted 23 of May 1920 at 6 P.M. o'clock. Delivered 25 of 1920 at 12.30 P.M. o'clock.

Warded of 19 at o'clock. Discharged undelivered of 19 at o'clock. by cause

	I. H.	I. M.	II. H.	II. M.	III. H.	III. M.	Total H.	Total M.
Duration of labour	29	-	1	30	2	30	32	-

Measurement of Pelvis—
Interspinous 23. Intercristal 26. Conj. ext. 19.5 Conj. diag. Conj. vera (estimated) Conj. vera (actual)

Abnormal conditions on admission—Discharges no Ulcers no Œdema no Catheter Urine no albumen

Presentation of Child Vertex Position of Child R.O.A.

Pains began date 23.5.20 hour 5 P.M. Rupture of membranes date 25.5.20 hour 11.30 A.M.
Delivery date 25.5.20 hour 12.30 P.M. (1) Spontaneous (2) Artificial

Operation or important complication

Hæmorrhage, amount Time of occurrence (a) Before (b) With (c) After Placenta
Source {Uterus / Lacerations} How arrested
Laceration {Cervix / Vagina / Perinæum {Through Sphincter / To Sphincter / Slight} / Labia} Union {Complete / Partial / None}

Placenta and membranes expelled—Complete Weight 1.2 ozs.
(a) Spontaneously. (b) By expression. (c) By hand introduced.
Chorion. (1) Intact. (2) Imperfect. (3) Retained.

Pulse. 80. On Admission. During second. After third.

INFANT. Male, female, weight, lb. 7 oz. 10 length, inches 20
3rd day " " 7 " 6
5th " " " 7 " 4
8th " " " 4 " 8
14th " " " "

Male, female, weight, lb. oz. length, inches
3rd day
5th
8th
14th

Born, alive, dead. Died before labour. Peeling. Macerated. Died during labour. Cause
Apparent age. Full Term Malformations,

Child's Head.	Names of all who Examined Patient.	Cord.
Circumference. 14	Physicians	Length 24 inches.
bi P. 3.6.	R.M.O.	Convolutions round child
bi.T. 3.2.	Labour Ward ~~Sister~~	Insertion
O.M. 5.2.	Pupil Midwives	Date of separation
O.F. 4.8.	Students	Condition of navel on leaving
S.O.F. 4.4.		Method of feeding
F.M. 2.		Condition of child on leaving Hospital
		Vaccination.—Date
		Result.

SPACE FOR BINDING.

FIG 3.7—*Detailed birth records kept at the Jessop Hospital, Sheffield, from 1907 onwards.*

fetal undernutrition in early gestation has profound and permanent effects on body size, undernutrition in late gestation has more profound effects on body proportion (page 18).

To be able to study the links between body proportions at birth and later death rates from coronary heart disease, a group of men and women born in the Jessop Hospital, Sheffield were traced. Since 1907 this hospital has kept unusually detailed records for each baby born there. At birth the baby was not only weighed but its length from crown to heel, head circumference, biparietal and other head diameters, and placental weight were recorded. In 1922 chest and abdominal circumference were added to this list of measurements. Fig 3.7 shows one of the records from the hospital. Not only was the baby measured in detail, but external measurements of the mother's pelvis were recorded, including the conjugate diameter, that is, the distance between the symphysis pubis and the fifth lumbar vertebra, and the intercristal diameter, that is, the distance between the iliac crests. The reason why such astonishingly detailed observations were made on each baby in this hospital and a number of others around Britain is not

TABLE 3.4—*Standardised mortality ratios according to birthweight and ponderal index at birth (birthweight/length³) among 1586 men born in Sheffield during 1907–23*

	Cause of death			
	All cardiovascular disease		Other causes	All causes
Variable measured	All ages	<65 years		
*Birthweight (lb)**				
≤5·5	119 (21)	125 (13)	118 (22)	118 (43)
−6·5	95 (61)	101 (34)	99 (67)	97 (128)
−7·5	105 (134)	111 (77)	101 (136)	103 (270)
−8·5	82 (730)	71 (36)	110 (103)	97 (176)
>8·5	74 (27)	68 (14)	127 (49)	101 (76)
All	94 (316)	94 (174)	107 (377)	101 (693)
Ponderal index (1000 × ounces/inches³)†				
≤12·5 (thinner babies)	113 (83)	118 (48)	105 (81)	109 (164)
−13·8	97 (78)	103 (45)	108 (91)	103 (169)
−15·1	86 (67)	89 (39)	110 (91)	98 (158)
>15·1 (fatter babies)	85 (66)	69 (29)	106 (87)	95 (153)
All	95 (294)	95 (161)	107 (350)	101 (644)

* 1 lb = 454 g.   †16 ounces = 1 lb. 1 inch = 2·54 cm. $1000 \times \dfrac{ounces}{inches^3} = \dfrac{1·732 \, kg}{m^3}$

Figures in parentheses are number of deaths.

known, although it seems that the record form was based on one devised at Queen Charlotte's Hospital in London.

Table 3.4 shows death rates among 1586 men born in the Jessop Hospital during 1907–23. Of the men 316 had died from cardiovascular disease; of these 235 were certified as resulting from coronary heart disease. Cardiovascular death rates fell with increasing birthweight. The ponderal index (birthweight/length³) of each baby was calculated. A low ponderal index is a standard indicator of thinness at birth. Table 3.4 shows that cardiovascular death rates fell from those men who were thin at birth to those who were fat, with a particularly marked trend for deaths before the age of 65 years. There were no similar trends in deaths from non-cardiovascular causes, although the cardiovascular disease trends were reflected in trends in deaths from all causes.

Men who had a small head circumference at birth also had raised death rates from cardiovascular disease. Those who had both a small head circumference (<14 inches) and a low ponderal index (≤13·8 ounces/inches³ × 1000) at birth had a standardised mortality ratio of 120 for premature cardiovascular deaths, compared with 75 in those who had a large head circumference (≥14 inches) and a high ponderal index (>13·8). Cardiovascular mortality was not related to the duration of gestation, except for a small increase in death rates among men born pre-term. The associations with thinness and head circumference at birth must therefore reflect associations with patterns of fetal growth.

47

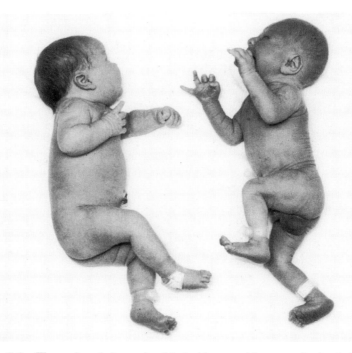

FIG 3.8—*The newborn baby on the right is thinner and has a smaller head circumference than the other baby.*

A thesis of this book, which is developed in later chapters, is that the baby with a small head circumference who is thin at birth was undernourished in mid-gestation.[56] Among the consequences are failure in the development of skeletal muscle, elevation of blood pressure (see chapter 4), and persistent disturbance of glucose/insulin metabolism (see chapter 6). Fig 3.8 shows such a baby. They tend to catch up in weight after birth.[78]

In addition to the association with thinness at birth, cardiovascular death rates were also raised in men who were short at birth with a crown:heel length of 20 inches or less ($\leqslant 50.8$ cm) although the difference was small and needs to be confirmed in other studies. Babies who are short and have reduced abdominal circumferences in relation to their head size are thought to have been undernourished in late gestation.[6] Among the consequences are failure of liver development, persistent elevation of blood pressure (see chapter 4) and disturbance of cholesterol metabolism and blood clotting (see chapter 5). Fig 3.9 shows such a baby. Their growth does not catch up in infancy. Thin and short babies seem to be vulnerable to coronary heart disease because of different metabolic abnormalities. Sex differences in the proportions of thin and short babies could explain the different

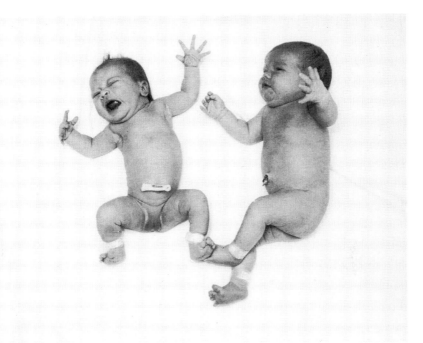

FIG 3.9—*The newborn baby on the left has a similar head circumference to the other baby but is shorter and has a smaller abdominal circumference.*

associations between weight at the age of one and cardiovascular disease in men and women. It has been suggested that boys are more vulnerable to undernutrition in late gestation because of their more rapid growth trajectory.[3 9 10] A disproportionate number of boys are therefore short at birth, and fail to gain weight in infancy, whereas girls tend to be thin at birth and their growth catches up in infancy. This hypothesis provides a framework within which the lower rates of cardiovascular disease in women than in men can be explored.

The average placental weight was 1·3 lb (591 g). Men who had the highest placental weight : birthweight ratio, with a ratio exceeding 0·215, had high death rates from cardiovascular disease. The standardised mortality ratio was 137, or 146 for premature deaths. The importance of a high placental weight : birthweight ratio in the prediction of cardiovascular disease first became apparent in studies of blood pressure, which are described in chapter 4. Disturbance of the placental weight : fetal weight ratio is thought to indicate fetal undernutrition (see chapter 9).

Studies of women in Sheffield are in progress. They have taken longer to complete than those of men, and the results are not yet known.

Intrauterine growth retardation and death from cardiovascular disease

The findings in Hertfordshire and Sheffield, and the findings described later in the book, show that the relationship between fetal growth and cardiovascular disease is continuous. Death rates fall progressively up to the highest values of birthweight and weight at one year of age. If the criteria for successful fetal growth are to include adult health and longevity, these findings reinforce the view that infants with significant intrauterine growth retardation need not necessarily be "light for gestational age".[11] Intrauterine growth retardation seems to be widespread, affecting many babies whose birthweights are within the normal range, not just those few who are recognised clinically by their unusually small size, and high risk of perinatal complications and death.

Confounding variables

These findings suggest that influences linked to early growth have an important effect on the risk of coronary heart disease and stroke. It may, however, be argued that people whose growth was impaired *in utero* and during infancy continue to be exposed to an adverse environment in childhood and adult life, and it is this later environment that produces the effects attributed to programming. The findings in this chapter, and in later chapters, which describe the links between early growth and cardiovascular risk factors such as blood pressure, point to five reasons why this argument cannot be sustained.

1. Associations between early growth and cardiovascular risk factors are being found in different populations. The association between low birthweight and cardiovascular disease has been shown in Hertfordshire and Sheffield. The association between low birthweight and impaired glucose tolerance in adults has been shown in three studies in Britain and two studies in the USA (see chapter 6). The association with raised blood pressure has been shown in four studies of adults, and is consistently found in children (see chapter 4).
2. In studies of blood pressure (see chapter 4), plasma fibrinogen and serum cholesterol concentrations (see chapter 5), and non-insulin dependent diabetes the associations with early growth are independent of social class at birth, social class as an adult, cigarette smoking, alcohol consumption, and obesity. Adult lifestyle, however, adds to the effects of early life. For example, the prevalence of impaired glucose tolerance is highest in people who had low birthweight but become obese as adults.
3. In studies of survivors in the Hertfordshire cohort, birthweight is unrelated to social class either at birth or currently.

4. The association between early weight and cardiovascular disease is specific. In neither women nor men were birthweight or weight at one year of age associated with death from lung cancer, which serves as an indicator of cigarette smoking, nor were they associated with deaths from all non-cardiovascular causes.

5. The associations are strong and graded. The association in men between cardiovascular death and weight at one year of age is remarkably strong and highly statistically significant. Body weight at birth is only a proxy for the changes in the body's structure, physiology, and metabolism which have been programmed *in utero*, and yet the relative risks associated with low birthweight are large: the risk of syndrome X (non-insulin dependent diabetes, hypertension, and hyperlipidaemia), for example, is ten times higher among men whose birthweight was 6·5 lb or less ($\leqslant 2·95$ kg) than among those whose birthweight was more than 9·5 lb (>4·32 kg).

It is reasonable to conclude from these points that reduced early growth and cardiovascular disease are causally linked. This conclusion is strengthened by recent animal studies which show, for example, that experimentally induced low birthweight is followed by persistently raised blood pressure.

Summary

In men and women, small size at birth is associated with raised death rates from cardiovascular disease in later life. The associations with small size at birth are independent of length of gestation and must therefore reflect low rates of fetal growth. Cardiovascular disease is not only linked to reduced fetal growth rates but to patterns of fetal growth that result in disproportionate body size, including thinness and shortness at birth. Cardiovascular disease in men, but not women, is also strongly associated with failure of weight gain during infancy, thought to be a consequence of undernutrition in late gestation, leading to failure of longitudinal growth in infancy. Reduced early growth is causally linked to cardiovascular disease in later life.

1 Acheson ED. Food policy, nutrition and government. The tenth Boyd Orr memorial lecture. *Proc Nutr Soc* 1986;**45**:131–8.
2 Barker DJP, Winter PD, Osmond C, Margetts B, Simmonds SJ. Weight in infancy and death from ischaemic heart disease. *Lancet* 1989;**ii**:577–80.
3 Osmond C, Barker DJP, Winter PD, Fall CHD, Simmonds SJ. Early growth and death from cardiovascular disease in women. *BMJ* 1993;**307**:1519–24.
4 Cox DR. Regression models and life-tables. *J R Stat Soc Ser B* 1972;**34**:187–220.
5 Robinson SM, Wheeler T, Hayes MC, Barker DJP, Osmond C. Fetal heart rate and intrauterine growth. *Br J Obstet Gynaecol* 1991;**98**:1223–7.

6 Barker DJP, Gluckman PD, Godfrey KM, Harding JE, Owens JA, Robinson JS. Fetal nutrition and cardiovascular disease in adult life. *Lancet* 1993;**341**:938–41.

7 Holmes GE, Miller HC, Hassanein K, Lansky SB, Goggin JE. Postnatal somatic growth in infants with atypical fetal growth patterns. *Am J Dis Child* 1977;**131**: 1078–83.

8 Villar J, Smeriglio V, Martorell R, Brown CH, Klein RE. Heterogenous growth and mental development of intrauterine growth retarded infants during the first 3 years of life. *Pediatrics* 1984;**74**:783–91.

9 Pedersen JF. Ultrasound evidence of sexual differences in fetal size in first trimester. *BMJ* 1980;**281**:1253.

10 Burgoyne PS. A Y-chromosomal effect on blastocyst cell numbers in mice. *Development* 1993;**117**:341–5.

11 Altman DG, Hytten FE. Intrauterine growth retardation: let's be clear about it. *Br J Obstet Gynaecol* 1989;**96**:1127–32.

4: Blood pressure

The association of reduced growth rates in fetal life and infancy with increased death rates from cardiovascular disease in adult life poses the question of what processes link the two. Raised blood pressure increases the risk of coronary heart disease and stroke. It is an obvious possible link between the intrauterine environment and these diseases because there is already good evidence that it originates in childhood.[1-3] The persistence of rank order of blood pressure among subjects examined at intervals—so called "tracking"—has been repeatedly observed in longitudinal studies of children as well as of adults.[4-8]

Fetal growth and adult blood pressure

The first suggestion that adult blood pressure may be related to fetal growth came from the study by Wadsworth and colleagues[9] of a national sample of people who were born in Britain during 1946, and followed up and examined at 36 years of age. Those with lower birthweights had higher systolic blood pressure. This observation has been confirmed in a re-analysis of the data and in three studies of middle aged men and women in Britain.[10-13] Table 4.1 shows mean systolic blood pressure in a group of men and women in Hertfordshire. The pressures fall progressively from those who weighed 5·5 lb or less ($\leqslant$2·5 kg) at birth to those who weighed

TABLE 4.1—*Mean systolic pressure in men and women aged 64–71 years, according to birthweight*

Birthweight (lb)*	Men	Women
$\leqslant$5·5	171 (18)	169 (9)
−6·5	168 (53)	165 (33)
−7·5	168 (144)	160 (68)
−8·5	165 (111)	163 (48)
>8·5	163 (92)	155 (26)
Total	166 (418)	161 (184)
s.d.	24	26
p (for trend)	0·02	0·1

*1 lb = 454 g.
Figures in parentheses are numbers of subjects.

more than 8·5 lb (>3·86 kg).[12] Diastolic pressure showed similar trends. As would be expected blood pressure was higher in people who were currently obese, as measured by the body mass index (weight/height^2). However, men and women who had lower birthweight had higher systolic pressure at any level of current body mass. (Although the trends in women are not statistically significant in table 4.1, other studies have shown equally strong and significant trends in men and women.)

Two other studies in Britain were carried out in Sheffield and Preston. The study in Sheffield was based on the detailed records kept at the Jessop Hospital for Women. Similarly detailed records were kept at Sharoe Green Hospital, in Preston. In both studies the association between low birthweight and raised blood pressure was shown to depend on babies who were small for dates, after reduced fetal growth, rather than on babies who were born pre-term. Although alcohol consumption and higher body mass were also associated with raised blood pressure, the associations between birthweight and blood pressure were independent of these influences.

As an alternative to a direct intrauterine influence on blood pressure, Ounsted and colleagues[14] have postulated that the accelerated growth of healthy babies of low birthweight during the first six months after birth might, of itself, accelerate the rise in blood pressure; the resultant above average values might persist.[14] Infant growth was recorded in the Hertfordshire data. Weight gain in infancy was not related to later blood pressure after making allowances for birthweight and current body size.[12] This suggests that high blood pressure is initiated pre- rather than postnatally. Raised blood pressure and catch up growth could, however, both be determined through growth failure *in utero*.

In the Sheffield and Preston studies, blood pressure in middle life could be related to body proportions at birth, as well as to birthweight. To examine the links between body proportions at birth and later blood pressure, babies born pre-term were excluded, because body proportions change during gestation. Analyses in Preston defined two groups of babies who developed raised blood pressures.[15 16] The first group were thin at birth, with a low ponderal index (birthweight/length^3) and a below average head circumference (see fig 3.8). The second had a short crown–heel length in relation to the head circumference, and therefore a high head circumference : length ratio (see fig 3.9). Short babies tend to be fat and may have above average birthweight.

The analyses in Preston revealed a difficulty that occurs when there are both thin and short babies in a study sample. Thin babies tend to have a low head circumference : length ratio, and short babies tend to be fat. The trends of raised blood pressure with low ponderal index and a high head circumference : length ratio therefore oppose each other. In the Preston data, however, thin babies had below average placental weight, whereas short babies had above average placental weight. Table 4.2 shows how

TABLE 4.2—*Mean systolic pressure of men and women aged 46–54, born after 38 completed weeks of gestation, according to ponderal index at birth and placental weight*

Placental weight (lb)*	Ponderal index ((ounces/inches³) × 1000)†				
	≤12	−13·25	−14·75	>14·75	All
≤1·25	154	147	142	141	147
	(53)	(54)	(42)	(25)	(174)
>1·25	148	149	152	154	152
	(27)	(27)	(48)	(50)	(152)
	152	148	147	150	149
All	(80)	(81)	(90)	(75)	(326)

*1 lb = 454 g. †16 ounces = 1 lb. 1 inch = 2·54 cm.
Figures in parentheses are numbers of subjects.

division of the data by placental weight revealed strong trends. At placental weights of 1·25 lb or less (≤591 g), a low ponderal index was associated with high adult blood pressure, the p value for the trend being 0·0001. At placental weights of more than 1·25 lb (>591 g), a high head circumference : length ratio was associated with high adult blood pressure, with $p = 0·02$.

The mean ponderal index of the babies in Sheffield was higher than that in Preston: fewer of the babies were thin.[13] Table 4.3 shows the strong association between birth length, abdominal circumference, and blood pressure. Babies who were short and had a small abdominal circumference at birth had the highest blood pressures as adults.

TABLE 4.3—*Mean systolic blood pressure, in men and women aged 50 years, according to length and abdominal circumference at birth*

Variable	Mean systolic pressure (mm Hg)*
Length (inches)†	
<20	151 (117)
−20	151 (114)
>20	142 (105)
All	148 (336)
p value for trend	0·001
Abdominal circumference (inches)†	
<11·5	154 (76)
−12·25	147 (74)
−13	149 (112)
>13	143 (71)
All	148 (333)
p value for trend	0·01

* Adjusted for sex, current body mass, alcohol intake, and gestational age.
†1 inch = 2·54 cm.
Figures in parentheses are numbers of subjects.

TABLE 4.4—*Mean systolic blood pressure by birthweight and current weight as fifths of their distributions in boys and girls, aged 5–7 years*

Birthweight (g)	Boys ($n=1789$); current weight (kg)					
	13·1–18·8	18·9–20·4	20·5–21·7	21·8–23·7	23·8–47·8	Mean (s.d.)
<3000	96·5	100·6	100·8	103·1	108·6	100·2 (9·0)
3000–	97·3	99·9	100·4	103·6	106·5	101·0 (8·6)
3290–	94·8	98·9	100·5	102·6	106·8	101·1 (9·2)
3530–	96·0	99·7	100·3	102·3	104·3	101·1 (8·5)
⩾3800	96·4	98·0	99·7	100·8	104·4	101·0 (8·0)
Mean (s.d.)	96·4 (8·3)	99·6 (7·6)	100·2 (7·7)	102·5 (8·2)	105·4 (8·7)	

Birthweight (g)	Girls ($n=1802$); current weight (kg)					
	13·3–18·1	18·2–20·0	20·1–21·4	21·5–23·6	23·7–47·0	Mean (s.d.)
<2820	97·7	99·7	102·6	105·3	105·5	101·1 (9·4)
2820–	97·7	100·1	100·8	102·0	107·8	101·0 (9·2)
3170–	94·5	97·7	100·6	103·2	103·7	100·0 (8·8)
3390–	96·6	99·0	99·7	102·4	105·8	101·0 (8·0)
⩾3660	95·6	97·9	98·9	99·5	104·5	100·4 (8·9)
Mean (s.d.)	96·8 (9·0)	98·9 (8·2)	100·4 (7·6)	102·1 (8·4)	105·2 (8·8)	

Fetal growth and blood pressure in children

The association between raised blood pressure and low birthweight is already apparent in childhood,[17–22] and is independent of the child's current size, although this is a powerful predictor of childhood blood pressure.[17 20] Two studies of teenagers have shown only weak associations between birthweight and blood pressure.[23 24] However, tracking of blood pressure is perturbed during the period of rapid growth in adolescence, which may provide an explanation. Table 4.4 shows systolic pressure by birthweight and current weight in 3591 boys and girls aged 5–7 years who were studied by Whincup.[21] At each birthweight, blood pressure rises from children who are light to those who are heavy. At each current weight, blood pressure falls from those who had low to those who had high birthweights. Children's weight indicates biological maturity: at any age a heavier, taller child is likely to be more biologically mature than a lighter, shorter child. Although blood pressure variation in childhood is dominated by differences in the rate of development, it is not known whether these differences establish patterns of blood pressure in adult life.

Table 4.5 shows findings from an unselected group of four-year-old children in Salisbury, England, the children being grouped according to ponderal index. Consistent with the findings in adults (see table 4.2), those who were thin at birth, having a low ponderal index, have higher systolic pressures after allowing for their current body size.[22]

TABLE 4.5—*Mean systolic blood pressure (adjusted for current weight and gestation) in children aged four years according to ponderal index at birth*

Ponderal index (kg/m³)	No. of children	Systolic pressure (mm Hg)
≤ 23·0	81	107
− 25·0	90	106
− 27·5	99	105
> 27·5	89	104

Amplification

Comparison of the results for adults and children in tables 4.1–5 shows that the differences in blood pressure in children are small compared with those in adults. The figure brings together the relationships between birthweight and blood pressure in all known studies of children and adults which include data on current body size. In fig 4.1, systolic pressure is regressed simultaneously on birthweight and either weight in children or body mass index in adults. The regression coefficients give the mean difference in systolic pressure per kilogram increase in birthweight. With the exception of a small study in Jamaica, an inverse relationship between birthweight and systolic pressure is apparent in pressure measurements made from the early months of life up to the age of 71 years. The strength of this relationship, however, increases progressively with age, as indicated by the size of the regression coefficient. Whereas in childhood a 1 kg increase in birthweight is equivalent to a fall in systolic pressure of 1–2 mm Hg, in adults the difference is around 5 mm Hg. The regression coefficients in adults remain larger than those in children, even after dividing them by the standard deviation to take account of the increase in standard deviation with age.

An interpretation of these findings is that differences in blood pressure are established *in utero*, but progressively amplified throughout life. The existence of initiating and amplification mechanisms in the aetiology of essential hypertension was first postulated by Folkow.[29] In patients with secondary hypertension from phaeochromocytoma, Conn's syndrome, or renal artery stenosis, hypertension may persist even after the initiating cause—the tumour or stenosis—has been removed.[30][31] There is, as yet, little evidence to show whether similar amplification processes, leading to persistence of raised blood pressure independent of initiating cause, occur in essential hypertension. The rise in blood pressure with increasing age is, however, consistent with this.

One can speculate on the mechanisms underlying initiation and amplification. The initiating process could be increased activity of a trophin or mitogen, leading to changes in the blood vessel wall and subsequent

BLOOD PRESSURE

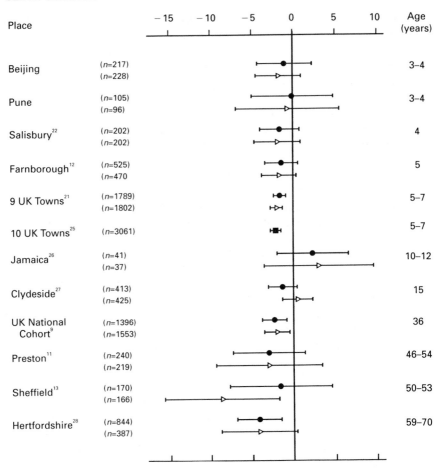

FIG 4.1—*Difference in systolic pressure (mm Hg) per kg of birthweight (adjusted for weight in children and body mass index in adults).* ● = *Males;* ▷ = *females;* ■ = *combined.*

rise in blood pressure. Possible trophins include growth hormone, insulin, insulin-like growth factor I (somatomedin C), cortisol, catecholamines, and angiotensin II.[31] A wide variety of endocrine changes has been shown in growth retarded fetal sheep.[32] Interest in the possible long-term effects of fetal exposure to glucocorticoids has been stimulated by the recent findings that treatment of pregnant rats with low dose dexamethasone leads to raised blood pressure in the adult offspring. The mechanisms underlying this are unclear but they may represent programming of fetal blood pressure by exposure to maternal steroids (page 27).

The feedback mechanism which amplifies the initiating effects with age could depend on progressive changes in the structure and elasticity of blood vessels. Experiments have shown that a short period of hypertension in young animals induces irreversible changes in the mechanical properties of the arterial wall.[33] In the growth retarded fetus there are changes in Doppler blood flow velocity waveforms in several vascular beds, including the descending aorta and cerebral vasculature.[34][35] These changes indicate selective modification of peripheral vascular resistance in the fetus which lead to the preferential perfusion of the brain at the expense of the trunk.

In babies born with a single umbilical artery, the iliac artery which gave rise to it is elastic whereas the other iliac artery, in which blood flow was lower, is thin walled and muscular. These differences in arterial structure persist. Measurements of arterial compliance in five-year-old children born with a single umbilical artery show that the iliac artery on the side of the single umbilical artery remains more elastic.[36] Arterial compliance determines pulse pressure, changes in which alter the scleroprotein content of the vessel wall; this, in turn, changes arterial compliance. In this way adaptations in the fetal pattern of circulation could alter the structure of blood vessels and perpetuate and amplify raised systolic blood pressure from infancy to old age.[37] In a group of 50-year-old men and women who were studied recently, those who were smaller at birth had reduced compliance in the femoral artery.[13] This supports the hypothesis that changes in the elasticity of vessel walls amplify initial elevations of blood pressure *in utero* through childhood into adult life.

Blood pressure of the mother

The blood pressures of the mothers of the men and women in the Sheffield study (see table 4.3) and the children in the Salisbury study (see table 4.5) were recorded.[13][22] In both studies, the associations between body size and proportions at birth and later blood pressure were independent of the mothers' blood pressures. In the Salisbury study, the blood pressures of the fathers were also measured and found to be related to those of the children. The relationship was, however, weaker than that with the mothers' systolic pressures. This has been found before and has been ascribed to X linked genes. Another possibility is that higher blood pressure in a mother reflects her own fetal experience, which, in turn, influences the intrauterine environment provided for her children. Studies of the Dutch Hunger Winter (page 122) have shown that women whose mothers were malnourished during pregnancy went on to have babies with retarded intrauterine growth. The effects of famine on the women's blood pressure are currently being studied.

Placental weight and blood pressure

Table 4.6 shows the systolic pressure of a group of men and women who were born, at term, in Sharoe Green Hospital in Preston, 50 years ago.[11][15] The subjects are grouped according to their birthweight and placental

TABLE 4.6—*Mean systolic blood pressure of men and women aged 50, born after 38 completed weeks of gestation, according to placental weight and birthweight*

Birthweight (lb)*	Placental weight (lb)				
	≤1·0	−1·25	−1·5	>1·5	All
−6·5	149 (24)	152 (46)	151 (18)	167 (6)	152 (94)
−7·5	139 (16)	148 (63)	146 (35)	159 (23)	148 (137)
>7·5	131 (3)	143 (23)	148 (30)	153 (40)	149 (96)
All	144 (43)	148 (132)	148 (83)	156 (69)	149† (327)

*1 lb = 454 g. †s.d. = 20·4.
Figures in parentheses are numbers of subjects.

weight. Consistent with findings in other studies systolic pressure fell from subjects with low to those with high birthweight. In addition, however, there was a hitherto unsuspected increase in blood pressure with increasing placental weight. Subjects with a mean systolic pressure of 150 mm Hg or more, a level sometimes used to define hypertension in clinical practice, comprised a group who as babies were relatively small in relation to the size of their placentas. There were similar trends with diastolic pressure. The differences in systolic pressure among all subjects, shown in the margin of table 4.6, are consistent with the difference in pressure of a few millimetres of mercury associated with 1 kg differences in birthweight found in other surveys of adults (see fig 4.1). As expected, birthweight and placental weight were strongly correlated (coefficient = 0·53). The fall in systolic pressure of 10 mm Hg, associated with increasing birthweight, is therefore statistically opposed by the rise of 12 mm Hg associated with increasing placental weight. These two large and independent trends are concealed when all pressures at a given birthweight are combined.

A rise in blood pressure with increasing placental weight was also found in four-year-old children in the Salisbury study.[22] In sheep and rats the placenta may enlarge in response to undernutrition in early pregnancy.[38 39] This is thought to be an adaptive response to increase the transfer of nutrients from the mother to her fetus. In humans, placental enlargement occurs in association with anaemia of pregnancy. Our limited knowledge of the nutritional control of placental growth is described in chapter 9.

The findings in table 4.6 suggest that maternal undernutrition increases the blood pressure of the offspring. Direct evidence comes from two studies. The systolic pressures of the children in the Salisbury study, whose mothers' haemoglobin in pregnancy fell below 10·0 g/dl, were 2·9 mm Hg higher than those of the other children.[22] Systolic pressure was also raised in Jamaican children whose mothers had thin skinfold thickness and low weight gain in pregnancy.[26]

TABLE 4.7—*Effect of fetal exposure to low protein on systolic pressure in adult rats*

Maternal protein intake during pregnancy (% by weight)	No. of animals	Systolic blood pressure (mm Hg)
18	15	137
12	13	152
9	13	153
6	11	159
p value for trend		<0·001

Animal experiments

Recent experiments on rats give direct evidence that blood pressure is linked to the mothers' nutrition in pregnancy. Female rats were given diets with differing protein content before mating and throughout pregnancy.[40] The diets were suboptimal rather than grossly deficient. Normal feeding was restored after birth, and the female offspring were allowed to develop normally. As would be expected, the rats on lower protein diets had lower weight gain during pregnancy. Table 4.7 shows the systolic pressures of the offspring nine weeks after birth. Offspring of all three groups of females fed on a low protein diet had significantly higher systolic pressure than the offspring of those on a normal 18% protein intake. These differences persisted to 21 weeks after birth, by which time the rats were mature. These observations also demonstrated that impaired nutrient supply during fetal development may have significant physiological consequences in later life, without major effects on birth size. The processes underlying the persistent elevation of blood pressure in these experiments are not known, but changes in the activity of angiotensin converting enzyme were observed.

Adult lifestyle and blood pressure

Although the customary explanation for differences in people's blood pressures is that they depend on the environment during adult life, these findings suggest that the intrauterine environment has a dominant effect. Birth measurements are associated with adult blood pressure, independent of current body weight or alcohol consumption. Research into the adult environment and hypertension has focused on salt.[41 42] A recent cross cultural study in 52 centres concluded that "lowering the daily intake of sodium from 170 mmol to 70 mmol corresponds to a 2 mm Hg reduction in systolic pressure".[42] This is a small effect compared with those associated with fetal growth. Differences such as those in table 4.6 may have large effects on death from cardiovascular disease. The available data suggest that lowering the distribution of blood pressure among a population by

10 mm Hg would correspond to a 30% reduction in total attributable mortality.[43]

Information on maternal smoking was collected for the study of four-year-old children in Salisbury.[22] Consistent with findings in other studies, the children's blood pressures were not related to whether or not their mothers smoked during pregnancy. Smoking is associated with reduced rather than increased placental weight, although the reduction in placental weight is less than the reduction in birthweight.

Blood pressure and fingerprints

Fingerprint patterns and the shape of the palm provide additional evidence that blood pressure originates *in utero*.[44] The patterns formed by the dermal ridges on the fingers reflect growth and development during early gestation and are established by week 19. Babies who are thin at birth tend to have "whorls", patterns of ridges thought to result from swollen finger pads in early gestation. Studies in India and England have shown that people with a whorl on one or more fingers have raised blood pressure in adult life. Similarly, babies who are short at birth in relation to their head size tend to have narrow palms, and adults with hands that are long in relation to their breadth have raised blood pressure.

Summary

Babies who are small for dates have raised systolic and diastolic pressure as children and adults. These associations are independent of the subjects' current body mass and alcohol consumption, and the mothers' blood pressures. Differences in blood pressure are established *in utero*, but are then progressively amplified throughout life. Blood pressure is associated with disproportionate placental growth in relation to fetal size, which is thought to indicate undernutrition of the fetus. Experiments in animals support the hypothesis that undernutrition in the mother leads to persistent elevation of blood pressure in the offspring.

1 Evans JG. The epidemiology of stroke. *Age Ageing* 1979;**8** (suppl):50–6.
2 Hoffman A. Blood pressure in childhood: an epidemiological approach to the aetiology of hypertension. *J Hypertens* 1984;**2**:232–8.
3 MacMahon S, Peto R, Cutler JA, *et al*. Blood pressure, stroke and coronary heart disease. Part 1, Prolonged differences in blood pressure: prospective observational studies corrected for the regressional dilution bias. *Lancet* 1990;**335**:765–74.
4 de Swiet M, Fayers P, Shinebourne EA. Blood pressure survey in a population of newborn infants. *BMJ* 1976;**ii**:9–11.

5 Beaglehole R, Salmond CE, Eyles, EF. A longitudinal study of blood pressure in Polynesian children. *Am J Epidemiol* 1977;**105**:87–9.

6 Clarke WR, Schrott HG, Leaverton PE, Connor WE, Lauer RM. Tracking of blood lipids and blood pressures in school age children: the Muscatine study. *Circulation* 1978;**58**:626–34.

7 Voors AW, Webber LS, Berenson GS. Time course studies of blood pressure in children: the Bogalusa heart study. *Am J Epidemiol* 1979;**109**:320–34.

8 Labarthe DR, Eissa M, Varas C. Childhood precursors of high blood pressure and elevated cholesterol. *Annu Rev Public Health* 1991;**12**:519–41.

9 Wadsworth MEJ, Cripps HA, Midwinter RE, Colley JRT. Blood pressure in a national birth cohort, at the age of 36 related to social and familial factors, smoking, and body mass. *BMJ* 1985;**291**:1534–8.

10 Barker DJP, Osmond C, Golding J, Kuh D, Wadsworth MEJ. Growth in utero, blood pressure in childhood and adult life, and mortality from cardiovascular disease. *BMJ* 1989;**298**:564–7.

11 Barker DJP, Bull AR, Osmond C, Simmonds SJ. Fetal and placental size and risk of hypertension in adult life. *BMJ* 1990;**301**:259–62.

12 Law CM, de Swiet M, Osmond C, Fayers PM, Barker DJP, Cruddas AM, Fall CHD. Initiation of hypertension in utero and its amplification throughout life. *BMJ* 1993;**306**:24–7.

13 Martyn CN, Barker DJP, Jespersen S, Greenwald S, Osmond C, Berry C. Growth in utero, adult blood pressure and arterial compliance. *Br Heart J* (in press).

14 Ounsted MK, Cockburn JM, Moar VA, Redman CWG. Factors associated with the blood pressures of children born to women who were hypertensive during pregnancy. *Arch Dis Child* 1985;**60**:631–5.

15 Barker DJP, Godfrey KM, Osmond C, Bull A. The relation of fetal length, ponderal index and head circumference to blood pressure and the risk of hypertension in adult life. *Paediatric and Perinatal Epidemiology* 1992;**6**:35–44.

16 Barker DJP, Gluckman PD, Godfrey KM, Harding JE, Owens JA, Robinson JS. Fetal nutrition and cardiovascular disease in adult life. *Lancet* 1993;**341**:938–41.

17 Voors AW, Webber LS, Frerichs RR, Berenson GS. Body height and body mass as determinants of basal blood pressure in children—the Bogalusa heart study. *Am J Epidemiol* 1977;**106**:101–8.

18 Simpson A, Mortimer JG, Silva PA, Spears G, Williams S. In: Onesi G, Kim KE, eds, *Hypertension in the young and old.* New York: Grune and Stratton, 1981:153–63.

19 Cater J, Gill M. The follow-up study: medical aspects. In: Illsey R, Mitchell RG, eds, *Low birthweight, a medical, psychological and social study.* Chichester: Wiley, 1984:191–205.

20 de Swiet M, Fayers P, Shinebourne E. Blood pressure in four and five year old children. The effects of environment and other factors in its measurement. *J Hypertens* 1984;**2**:501–5.

21 Whincup PH, Cook DG, Shaper AG. Early influences on blood pressure: a study of children aged 5–7 years. *BMJ* 1989;**299**:587–91.

22 Law CM, Barker DJP, Bull AR, Osmond C. Maternal and fetal influences on blood pressure. *Arch Dis Child* 1991;**66**:1291–5.

23 Seidman DS, Laor A, Gale R, Stevenson DK, Mashiach S, Danon YL. Birthweight, current body weight and blood pressure in late adolescence. *BMJ* 1991;**302**:1235–7.

24 Williams S, St George IM, Silva PA. Intrauterine growth retardation and blood pressure at age seven and eighteen. *J Clin Epidemiol* 1992;**45**:1257–73.

25 Whincup PH, Cook DG, Papacosta O. Do maternal and intrauterine factors influence blood pressure in childhood? *Arch Dis Child* 1992;**67**:1423–9.

26 Godfrey KM, Forrester T, Barker DJP, *et al.* Maternal nutritional status in pregnancy and blood pressure in childhood. *Br J Obstet Gynaecol* 1994;**101**:398–403.

27 Macintyre S, Watt G, West P, Ecob R. Correlates of blood pressure in 15 year olds in the West of Scotland. *J Epidemiol Community Health* 1991;**45**:143–7.

28 Hales CN, Barker DJP, Clark PMS, *et al.* Fetal and infant growth and impaired glucose tolerance at age 64. *BMJ* 1991;**303**:1019–22.

29 Folkow B. Cardiovascular structural adaptation: its role in the initiation and maintenance of primary hypertension. *Clin Sci* 1978;**55**(suppl):3–22.

30 Ferris J, Brown J, Fraser R, *et al.* Results of adrenal surgery in patients with hypertension, aldosterone excess and low plasma renin concentration. *BMJ* 1975;**i**: 135–8.

31 Lever A, Harrap S. Essential hypertension: a disorder of growth with origins in childhood. *J Hypertens* 1992;**10**:101–20.

32 Owens J, Owens P, Robinson J. Experimental fetal growth retardation: metabolic and endocrine aspects. In: Gluckman PD, Johnston BM, Nathanielsz PW, eds, *Advances in fetal physiology.* Ithaca, NY: Perinatalogy Press, 1989:263–86.

33 Berry CL, Greenwald SE. Effects of hypertension on the static mechanical properties and chemical composition of the rat aorta. *Cardiovasc Res* 1976;**10**:437–51.

34 Al-Ghazali W, Chita SK, Chapman MG, Allan LD. Evidence of redistribution of cardiac output in asymmetrical growth retardation. *Br J Obstet Gynaecol* 1989;**96**: 697–704.

35 Wright JS, Cruickshank JK, Kontis S, Doré C, Gosling RG. Aortic compliance measured by non-invasive Doppler ultrasound: description of a method and its reproducibility. *Clin Sci* 1990;**78**:463–8.

36 Berry CL, Gosling RG, Laogun AA, Bryan E. Anomalous iliac compliance in children with a single umbilical artery. *Br Heart J* 1976;**38**:510–5.

37 Folkow B. Physiological aspects of primary hypertension. *Physiol Rev* 1982;**62**:347–504.

38 McCrabb GJ, Egan AR, Hosking BJ. Maternal undernutrition during mid-pregnancy in sheep. Placental size and its relationship to calcium transfer during late pregnancy. *Br J Nutr* 1991;**65**:157–68.

39 Levy L, Jackson AA. Modest restriction of dietary protein during pregnancy in the rat: fetal and placental growth. *J Dev Physiol* 1993;**19**:113–18.

40 Langley SC, Jackson AA. Increased systolic blood pressure in adult rats induced by fetal exposure to maternal low protein diets. *Clin Sci* 1994;**86**:217–22.

41 Anonymous. Diet and hypertension [Editorial]. *Lancet* 1984;**ii**:671–3.

42 Intersalt Cooperative Research Group. Intersalt: an international study of electrolyte excretion and blood pressure. Results for 24 hour urinary sodium and potassium excretion. *BMJ* 1988;**297**:319–28.

43 Rose G. Sick individuals and sick populations. *Int J Epidemiol* 1985;**14**:32.

44 Godfrey KM, Barker DJP, Peace J, Cloke J, Osmond C. Relation of fingerprints and shape of the palm to fetal growth and adult blood pressure. *BMJ* 1993;**307**:405–9.

5: Cholesterol and blood clotting

Serum cholesterol

The reasons why serum cholesterol concentrations differ among populations and among people within populations are not understood. They are important because cholesterol may be directly involved in the pathogenesis of atheroma and is strongly associated with the risk of coronary heart disease.[1][2] Cholesterol and triglycerides are the lipids of central importance in the development of atheroma and coronary heart disease. They are transported in the blood as lipoprotein complexes, which are classified into low density lipoproteins (LDLs) and high density lipoproteins (HDLs). Around 65% of the serum total cholesterol is carried in the LDL fraction and 25% in the HDL fraction. Raised LDL concentrations are associated with an increased risk of coronary heart disease, whereas raised HDL concentrations seem to be protective.

Chapter 2 gave an account of animal experiments in which lipid metabolism was permanently changed by interference with diet, and other manipulations during gestation and shortly after birth. Speculation that the high cholesterol and saturated fat content of human milk influence lipid metabolism throughout life has not been supported by animal experiments or follow up studies of children. The concentration of cholesterol in infant food seems to have only a transient effect on serum cholesterol concentrations. Animal studies unequivocally demonstrate, however, that interference with cholesterol metabolism during development affects lipid metabolism permanently. This chapter describes early evidence that similar phenomena occur in humans.

Fetal growth and adult serum cholesterol concentrations

At the Jessop Hospital for Women in Sheffield, measurements of the babies' body size at birth were unusually detailed (see fig 7 in chapter 3). They included not only birthweight, length, and head circumference, but abdominal and chest circumferences. Out of 1039 singleton infants born in the hospital during 1939–40, there were 219 who still lived in Sheffield and agreed to take part in a study which included measurement of fasting serum lipid concentrations.[3]

Serum concentrations of total cholesterol, LDL cholesterol, and apo-lipoprotein B—the structural apolipoprotein linked to LDL cholesterol—tended to be higher in men and women with lower birthweight, although this was a weak association. The striking association was with a specific pattern of disproportionate growth, leading to a small abdominal cir-cumference at birth. Table 5.1 shows that the serum concentration of the three lipids fell from men and women whose abdominal circumference was 11·5 inches or less (≤29 cm) at birth to those whose abdominal circumference was more than 13 inches (>33 cm). The statistical sig-nificance of these trends was increased by adjustment for length of gestation. The figure 5.1 shows the values of LDL cholesterol for each of the 189 men and women with known gestation and abdominal circumference. In a simultaneous analysis with abdominal circumference, no other birth measurement was related to lipid concentration.

In table 5.2 the men and women are divided into five groups according to current body mass index. The weak, statistically non-significant trends in serum LDL cholesterol concentrations with current body mass contrast with the strong trends with abdominal circumference (see table 5.1). This is particularly remarkable because abdominal circumference was part of a series of routine measurements at birth and is therefore liable to error. The differences in serum cholesterol concentrations associated with the range of abdominal circumference at birth are clinically significant. Lowering serum cholesterol concentrations from 6·5 to 6·0 mmol/1 has been estimated to reduce risk of coronary heart disease by 30%.[4] The differences associated with abdominal circumference are at least as great as this.

Cigarette smoking and alcohol consumption were associated with higher serum concentrations of total and LDL cholesterol, and apolipoprotein B, but adjusting for these aspects of adult lifestyle strengthened the association between serum lipid concentrations and abdominal circumference at birth. Serum lipid concentrations did not differ by social class, either currently or at birth, and the association with abdominal circumference occurred within each social class group. In this study serum concentrations of HDL cholesterol and triglycerides showed no significant trends with any measurements at birth.

As was described in chapter 2 undernutrition in early intrauterine life tends to produce small but normally proportioned animals, whereas un-dernutrition later in development leads to selective organ damage and disproportionate growth.[5] During periods of undernutrition, those tissues that are more mature have a greater priority of growth, and may continue to grow at the expense of other tissues. The timing of undernutrition therefore determines which tissues and systems are selectively damaged, and hence the pattern of disproportion in organ size at birth.

TABLE 5.1—*Mean serum lipid concentrations according to abdominal circumference at birth in men and women aged 50–53 years*

Abdominal circumference (inches)*	No. of people		Total cholesterol (mmol/l)			LDL cholesterol (mmol/l)			Apolipoprotein B (g/l)		
	Men	Women	Men	Women	All	Men	Women	All	Men	Women	All
≤11·5	28	25	6·5	6·8	6·7	4·5	4·6	4·5	0·96	0·99	0·97
−12·0	22	21	6·8	6·9	6·9	4·8	4·4	4·6	0·95	0·97	0·96
−12·5	13	18	6·7	6·8	6·8	4·6	4·2	4·4	0·99	0·97	0·98
−13·0	21	24	6·0	6·5	6·2	3·8	4·2	4·0	0·90	0·93	0·91
>13·0	26	19	6·0	6·4	6·1	3·9	4·1	4·0	0·87	0·88	0·87
Total=/average	110	107	6·4	6·7	6·5	4·3	4·3	4·3	0·93	0·95	0·94
p value adjusted for gestational age by regression			0·009	0·16	0·003	0·003	0·12	0·0007	0·01	0·07	0·002†

*1 inch = 2·54 cm.
†Adjusted for body mass index.

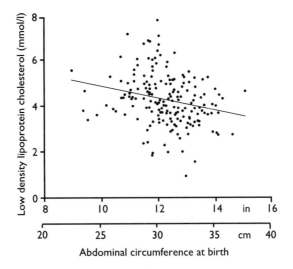

FIG 5.1—*Low density lipoprotein cholesterol concentrations plotted against abdominal circumference at birth, adjusted for duration of gestation in men and women aged 50–53 years.*

TABLE 5.2—*Mean serum low density lipoprotein concentrations according to current body mass index in men and women aged 50–53 years*

Current body mass index (kg/m²)	Men	Women
≤23	4·0 (14)	4·1 (17)
−25	4·5 (19)	4·4 (32)
−27	4·5 (30)	4·0 (20)
−30	4·1 (30)	4·8 (15)
>30	4·1 (17)	4·3 (23)
All	4·3 (110)	4·3 (107)

Figures in parentheses are numbers of subjects.

In late gestation the human fetus may respond to nutrient deprivation by sustaining the brain at the expense of trunk growth.[6] The liver, which is growing rapidly at this time, may be particularly compromised and its weight at birth is found to be low when compared with either the weight of the brain or total body weight.[7] During ultrasonography of the fetus, the head circumference : abdominal circumference ratio is used as a measure of the ratio of brain : liver size in disproportionate growth of this kind.[8] The association of serum total and LDL cholesterol concentrations with low abdominal circumference, but not independently with low head circumference, suggests that raised concentrations of these lipids in adult life are related to growth failure in late gestation. In the Sheffield study, chest circumference at birth did not predict serum lipid concentrations independently of abdominal circumference, which points to a specific association with growth failure of abdominal viscera, including the liver, rather than failure of growth of the trunk as a whole.

One possible explanation of these findings is that impaired growth of the liver in late gestation leads to permanent changes in LDL cholesterol metabolism. The liver is thought to be the major site for synthesis of LDL cholesterol in late gestation, and the human fetus requires large quantities at this time to sustain metabolic activities, which include high rates of secretion of steroid hormones by the adrenal glands.[9] Just before birth, rates of cholesterol synthesis in the liver, as judged by the activity of the rate limiting enzyme in cholesterol synthesis, are more than twice those in the adult.[10] Babies who are small for their gestational age have been reported to have raised serum LDL concentrations.[11] Follow up studies of children have shown that they maintain their rank order by serum cholesterol concentrations from the age of six months.[12 13]

The processes by which impaired liver growth in late gestation could lead, paradoxically, to persistently raised serum concentrations of LDL cholesterol are unknown. A study of LDL metabolism in samples of middle aged men in five countries has, however, led to the suggestion that differences in serum concentrations depend on different activity of LDL receptors in the liver.[14] Persistent reduction of LDL receptor activity, associated with failure of fetal liver growth, is one possible explanation for persisting elevation of serum cholesterol concentrations.

Infant feeding and adult serum cholesterol concentrations

During analyses of death from cardiovascular disease in Hertfordshire, which were described in chapter 3, death rates were found to differ according to the method of infant feeding.[15 16] When the health visitors in Hertfordshire visited the babies during infancy, they recorded how each baby was being fed. In the period up to 1930, 66% of the babies were

TABLE 5.3—*Standardised mortality ratios from cardiovascular disease below 65 years according to method of infant feeding*

Infant feeding	Men			Women		
	Standardised mortality ratio	(95% confidence interval)	No. of deaths	Standardised mortality ratio	(95% confidence interval)	No. of deaths
Breast and bottle fed	73	(63–82)	213	65	(47–89)	40
Breast fed, weaned before 1 year	72	(64–79)	377	65	(51–82)	73
Breast fed, not weaned at 1 year	93	(80–107)	181	63	(39–98)	20
Bottle fed only	81	(62–103)	64	108	(60–178)	15

recorded as breast fed, 27% as breast and bottle fed, and 7% as exclusively bottle fed. When the infants were one year old a record was made of whether or not they had been weaned. The term "weaned" can imply that either breast feeding has stopped or solid food has been introduced. The evidence from the Hertfordshire Chief Health Visitor's annual reports, together with anecdotal evidence from health visitors who worked in Hertfordshire around this period, suggest that "weaned" usually meant cessation of breast feeding. In her annual reports, Miss Burnside, the Chief Health Visitor for Hertfordshire, quoted percentages of breast fed babies weaned at 12 months, but gave no comparable information for bottle fed babies, presumably because the word did not usually apply.[17] In England, at the beginning of the century breast feeding was continued for longer than is now usual, but was commonly stopped at around nine months and usually before one year.[18 19] Around 20% of the babies in Hertfordshire were, however, breast fed beyond a year, and these babies tended to be from poorer families. Anecdotal evidence from Hertfordshire suggests that women in lower socioeconomic groups prolonged breast feeding beyond one year as a form of contraception.

It was surprising to find that death rates from cardiovascular disease were higher in two groups of people: those who had been breast fed beyond one year and those who had been exclusively bottle fed. Table 5.3 shows that raised death rates were found only in men who had been breast fed beyond one year, and not in women, whereas both men and women who had been exclusively bottle fed had raised rates, although this was not statistically significant. There were no important differences in mortality from non-cardiovascular causes in relation to the method of infant feeding.

TABLE 5.4—*Mean serum lipid concentrations in men aged 59–70 years according to infant feeding*

	Breast and bottle fed (1)	Breast fed, weaned before one year (2)	Breast fed, not weaned at one year (3)	Bottle fed only (4)	All	s.d.
Cholesterol (mmol/l)	6·6	6·6	6·9*	7·0*	6·7	1·2
Non-fasting cholesterol (mmol/l)	6·4	6·4	6·9**	7·1**	6·5	1·2
LDL cholesterol (mmol/l)	4·6	4·6	5·0**	5·1*	4·7	1·1
HDL cholesterol (mmol/l)	1·2	1·2	1·2	1·2	1·2	0·3
LDL : HDL ratio	3·8	3·8	4·2**	4·2	3·9	1·5
Triglyceride (mmol/l)	1·4	1·4	1·5	1·4	1·4	1·6
Apolipoprotein A1 (g/l)	1·31	1·30	1·29	1·35	1·30	1·2
Apolipoprotein B (g/l)	1·08	1·08	1·14	1·14	1·09	1·3
Number of men	116	253	91	25	485	

*$p<0·05$ **$p<0·01$. Comparison with groups (1) and (2) combined.

Fall and colleagues[15] measured the serum lipids in a sample of men who still lived in Hertfordshire. Table 5.4 shows that men who had been breast fed beyond one year, and those who had been exclusively bottle fed, had higher serum concentrations of total cholesterol in fasting and non-fasting samples, higher concentrations of LDL cholesterol, and higher LDL : HDL cholesterol ratios than men in the other two feeding groups.

There were no differences between infant feeding groups for other cardiovascular risk factors, including body mass, blood pressure, plasma glucose, insulin, fibrinogen, and factor VII concentrations. The percentages of men who were either current smokers or in social class IV or V were similar in all the feeding groups. In spite of the similarity in current social class, a higher percentage of men who had been breast fed beyond one year had been born into families of social class IV or V. Table 5.5 shows, however, that the higher concentrations of LDL cholesterol in these men were found in each social class. Findings for total cholesterol and apolipoprotein B were similar.

These findings suggest that, in men born 70 years ago who were breast fed and weaned relatively late, a process was established which led to raised serum concentrations of LDL cholesterol and increased death rates from coronary heart disease in adult life. This process was not linked to other lipids or other cardiovascular risk factors. The regulation of serum lipid

TABLE 5.5—*Mean serum LDL cholesterol concentration (mmol/l) in men aged 59–70 years according to infant feeding and social class at birth*

Social class at birth	Breast and bottle fed	Breast fed, weaned before one year	Breast fed, not weaned at one year	Bottle fed only	All groups	Standard deviation
I, II, III (non-manual)	4·8	4·6	5·1	4·9	4·7 (62)	1·0
III (manual)	4·5	4·7	5·0	5·6	4·7 (157)	1·1
IV, V	4·6	4·6	5·0	5·0	4·7 (225)	1·2
All classes	4·6	4·6	5·0	5·2	4·7 (444)	1·1

Figures in parentheses are numbers of men.

concentrations involves several tissues, most importantly the liver and gut. Mechanisms by which late weaning of infants might program lipid metabolism in adults are a matter for speculation. Breast milk contains several hormones and growth factors which can influence lipid metabolism, including thyroid hormones and steroids.[20][21] One possible explanation of the findings, which derives from observations on baboons, is that thyroid hormones present in breast milk may down regulate the suckling infant's thyroid function in later life, thereby influencing cholesterol metabolism.[22][23]

Breast milk provides ideal nourishment for the young infant, but there is evidence that some babies who are exclusively breast fed after six months receive inadequate energy.[24] Human breast milk contains low iron concentrations, and exclusively breast fed babies commonly develop low iron stores in the second half of infancy.[25] Breast milk may also be deficient in vitamins, notably vitamin D, if the mother is poorly nourished.[26] In Hertfordshire infants who were breast fed beyond one year weighed less and had fewer teeth at one year of age than those who were weaned. This may be evidence of poorer nutrition in the non-weaned group, although we cannot say whether these differences were the result of late weaning or a cause of it. Among men who were breast fed beyond one year, it was those with higher birthweights, but lower weights at one year of age, who had highest death rates from coronary heart disease.[15] They also had higher serum total and LDL cholesterol concentrations. One interpretation of this is that larger babies tended to outgrow an inadequate supply of nutrients.

The men and women who had been exclusively bottle fed, comprising only 7% of the sample, also had raised death rates from coronary heart disease and, at least in men, higher serum LDL cholesterol concentrations. We do not know what was contained in the bottle feeds because this was not specified in the Hertfordshire records. Bottle feeds available 70 years ago included patent preparations of dried cows' milk, unmodified cows' milk, diluted condensed milk, and patent foods made from wheatflour or arrowroot.[27] Modern formula milks differ from these foods: they are fortified with iron and vitamins; the fat content is mainly unsaturated; and the electrolyte content is similar to that of breast milk. It is therefore difficult to assess the relevance of these findings for bottle fed babies today. They do, however, add to the evidence that, in humans, as in animals, nutrition during infancy may have a permanent influence on lipid metabolism and the risk of coronary heart disease. A recent study in Croatia has added further evidence; young men and women breast fed for less than three months after birth had higher serum cholesterol concentrations than those breast fed for longer.[28]

Blood clotting

After the Second World War, research into coronary heart disease centred almost exclusively on atheroma and, because of its lipid content, the role of dietary fat and serum cholesterol concentrations. The role of blood clotting, though implied in the term "coronary thrombosis", was until recently overlooked. In 1951 Morris[29] drew attention to the probable role of processes other than atheroma in the genesis of coronary heart disease. Analysing postmortem findings at the London Hospital from the early years of this century, he showed that the prevalence of advanced atheroma had remained unchanged over a period of time in which mortality from coronary heart disease had increased several-fold. Clearly processes other than atheroma were involved in this steep rise. Interest in the role of thrombosis re-emerged when it was shown that thrombosis in the coronary vessels often preceded myocardial infarction and sudden coronary death.[30 31]

During the evolution of a thrombus, platelets adhere rapidly to damaged endothelium and each other. Thereafter fibrin becomes incorporated into the clot, giving it stability and volume. The importance of plasma concentrations of fibrinogen, the precursor of fibrin, as a predictor of death was first shown by Meade and colleagues in the Northwick Park Heart Study.[32 33] Men with high plasma concentrations of fibrinogen were shown to be at increased risk of myocardial infarction. Raised plasma levels of factor VII activity, part of the "extrinsic" pathway of the coagulation cascade involved in the production of thrombin, were also found to be associated with increased risk. Raised concentrations of fibrinogen and factor VII predispose to thrombosis, and may contribute to the development and progression of atheroma.[34]

Other studies have confirmed strong relationships between fibrinogen and coronary heart disease and stroke.[35-38] The association of coronary heart disease with fibrinogen is at least as strong as that with cholesterol.[33] Fibrinogen is an acute phase protein and rises in response to several stimuli.[39] Plasma concentrations are increased by cigarette smoking and much of the relationship between smoking and coronary heart disease may be mediated through this effect.[34] Factor VII activity is increased by eating fat, and dietary fat may therefore increase the risk of coronary heart disease through an immediate effect on thrombosis as well as a long term effect on atheroma.[40 41]

TABLE 5.6—*Mean plasma fibrinogen and factor VII concentrations in men aged 59–70 years according to weight at one year and birthweight*

Weight (lb)*	Number of men	Fibrinogen (g/l)	Factor VII (% of standard)
Weight at one year			
≤18	38	3·21	122
−20	93	3·10	111
−22	178	3·13	108
−24	173	2·97	106
−26	82	2·93	106
>26	33	2·93	103
p value for trend		<0·001	<0·005
Birthweight			
≤5·5	21	3·18	118
−6·5	70	3·06	104
−7·5	187	3·10	108
−8·5	183	2·98	107
−9·5	96	3·00	112
>9·5	40	3·05	109
p value for trend		0·10	0·84
All	597	3·04	108
s.d.		0·59	27

*1 lb = 454 g.

Fetal and infant growth and adult haemostatic factors

Table 5.6 shows mean plasma fibrinogen and factor VII concentrations in a sample of men in Hertfordshire.[42] Concentrations of both factors fell from those who had low to those who had high weight at one year; these trends were strongly statistically significant. Neither factor showed a significant trend with birthweight, although the highest concentrations of each were found in men with birthweights of 5·5 lb or less (≤2·5 kg). The difference in plasma fibrinogen concentrations between men who weighed 27 lb or more (≥12·3 kg) and those who weighed 18 lb or less (≤8·2 kg) at one year is statistically equivalent to an increase in the cardiovascular death rate of around 40%.[33]

When the men were grouped into current smokers, ex-smokers, and those who had never smoked, mean plasma fibrinogen concentrations were, as expected, highest in smokers; they were also higher in ex-smokers than in men who had never smoked (table 5.7). Adjustments for smoking did not change the correlation of mean plasma fibrinogen concentrations with weight at one year. Regression analysis showed that the concentration fell with increasing weight at one year in each smoking group. Table 5.7 provides an example of the adverse effects of adult lifestyle adding to those associated with failure of early growth. The highest plasma fibrinogen concentrations were in those men who had the lowest weight at one year

TABLE 5.7—*Mean plasma fibrinogen concentrations (g/l) in men aged 59–70 years according to their weight at one year of age and smoking habits*

Weight at one year (lb)*	Non-smokers	Ex-smokers	Current smokers
≤18	2·87 (6)	3·25 (19)	3·33 (12)
−20	3·25 (11)	2·94 (48)	3·28 (31)
−22	2·98 (31)	3·10 (96)	3·29 (50)
−24	2·81 (32)	2·95 (97)	3·14 (42)
−26	2·78 (16)	2·93 (46)	3·05 (18)
>26	2·62 (4)	3·00 (22)	2·87 (7)
All	2·90 (100)	3·01 (328)	3·20 (160)

Numbers of men in parentheses.
*1 lb = 454 g.

and smoked. The lowest concentrations were in those men who had the highest weight at one year and never smoked.

An analysis of plasma fibrinogen concentrations in the Preston sample of men (page 54), whose size at birth had been measured in detail, showed that those who were short at birth, having a low crown–heel length, had raised concentrations. This finding was subsequently confirmed in men and women in Sheffield, where men with low birthweight, short length, and reduced abdominal circumference at birth were found to have raised plasma fibrinogen concentrations. Table 5.8 shows the trend with abdominal circumference, which was strengthened after adjustment for the current waist : hip circumference ratio of the subjects. A high waist : hip ratio is independently associated with raised plasma fibrinogen concentrations.[42] Plasma fibrinogen concentrations among women were not linked to measurements at birth in Hertfordshire, Preston, or Sheffield. Little is known about the association between plasma fibrinogen and cardiovascular disease in women.[38] In the Framingham study[36] plasma fibrinogen was linked to coronary heart disease in younger women but not to stroke.

The associations between the two haemostatic factors and failure of early growth were independent of smoking, social class, alcohol consumption, and adult body mass; it does not seem possible to sustain the argument

TABLE 5.8—*Mean plasma fibrinogen concentrations (g/l) in men aged 50–53 years according to abdominal circumference at birth*

Abdominal circumference (inches)*	Unadjusted	Adjusted for smoking and waist:hip ratio	No. of men
≤11·5	2·60	2·66	25
−12·25	2·53	2·51	22
−13	2·49	2·47	35
>13	2·37	2·36	22
p value for trend	0·03	0·006	

*1 inch = 2·54 cm.

TABLE 5.9—*Mean plasma fibrinogen concentration in men aged 46–54 years according to ratio of placental weight : birthweight*

Placental weight : birthweight	Mean plasma fibrinogen concn (g/l)	No. of men
≤0·162	2·87	28
−0·182	2·89	30
−0·200	2·92	27
−0·229	2·90	28
>0·229	3·15	29
All	2·94	142
s.d.	0·50	

that the associations merely reflect the effects of confounding variables linked to both early growth failure and adult lifestyle.[42] Rather, these results suggest that there is a critical period in early life when the metabolism of haemostatic factors is programmed. Plasma concentrations of fibrinogen and factor VII are known to reach values within the adult range by the age of one year.[43]

Relative failure of growth in infancy, which is a strong predictor of fibrinogen and factor VII concentrations (see table 5.6), may result from either postnatal or prenatal influences; postnatal influences include feeding and illness. In Hertfordshire, where postnatal development was recorded, concentrations of the haemostatic factors did not vary in relation to differences in infant feeding and weaning, although these differences were related to adult cholesterol concentrations (see table 5.4). They were also not related to illness during infancy, although illness was related to adult lung function (see chapter 7). The findings in Preston and Sheffield (see table 5.8) suggest that prenatal influences may underlie the reduction in infant growth which is associated with high concentrations of the factors. The babies who subsequently have raised concentrations tend to be short at birth with a reduced abdominal circumference. As already described, the human fetus may respond to nutrient deprivation in late gestation by sustaining the brain at the expense of trunk growth;[6] the liver may be particularly compromised. After birth the growth of these babies, who tend to be short at birth, does not "catch up".[44][45] High adult concentrations of haemostatic factors could be associated with infant growth failure through a common origin in fetal undernutrition during late gestation. Table 5.9 shows that mean plasma fibrinogen concentrations among men in Preston rose progressively as the placental weight : birthweight ratio increased. As already described (page 60) a high placental weight : birthweight ratio is thought to indicate fetal undernutrition.

Circulating fibrinogen and factor VII concentrations are largely regulated by the liver. High adult concentrations may be a persistent response to impaired liver development during a critical early phase. One possibility, discussed further in chapter 9, is that one aspect of this impaired liver development could be its sensitivity to growth hormone and production of insulin-like growth factor I. Consistent with this, both fibrinogen and factor VII concentrations are linked to adult height, being lower in taller men.[42] It is interesting that when concentrations of either factor are simultaneously regressed with adult height and weight at one year of age, the association with adult height is abolished whereas that with infant weight remains—further evidence of the importance of early life. An inverse relationship between height and cardiovascular disease has been found in prospective studies of at least three populations: 1·8 million people in Norway who attended for mass radiography, 17 000 male civil servants in London, and 1700 men in Finland.[46–48]

Although raised concentrations of fibrinogen and factor VII may both reflect impaired liver development *in utero*, the underlying mechanisms may be different. Fibrinogen and factor VII concentrations are only weakly associated and, although fibrinogen concentrations are strongly related to blood pressure, factor VII concentrations are not.[41 42]

Summary

Animal studies show that interference with cholesterol metabolism during development, and breast feeding, permanently change lipid metabolism. There is now evidence that similar phenomena occur in humans. Raised serum concentrations of total and LDL cholesterol are found in men and women who had reduced liver size at birth, as measured by abdominal circumference. This suggests that impaired liver growth in late gestation may bring about a permanent alteration of LDL cholesterol metabolism. Raised LDL cholesterol concentrations and an increased risk of coronary heart disease are also found in men who had been breast fed for more than a year. This may reflect prolonged exposure to maternal hormones in breast milk.

Raised plasma concentrations of two haemostatic factors— fibrinogen and factor VII—are associated with an increased risk of cardiovascular disease. Raised concentrations of these factors are found in men who, at birth, were short with reduced abdominal circumferences, and who failed to gain weight in infancy. Circulating fibrinogen and factor VII concentrations are largely regulated by the liver. Impaired liver development during late gestation may program higher plasma concentrations in later life.

1 Keys A. *Seven countries*. Cambridge, MA: Harvard University Press, 1980.
2 Lewis B. The lipoproteins: predictors, protectors and pathogens. *BMJ* 1983;**287**: 1161–4.
3 Barker DJP, Martyn CN, Osmond C, Hales CN, Fall CHD. Growth in utero and serum cholesterol concentrations in adult life. *BMJ* 1993;**307**:1524–7.
4 Wald NJ. Cholesterol and coronary heart disease: to screen or not to screen. In: Marmot M, Elliott P, eds, *Coronary heart disease epidemiology*. Oxford: Oxford University Press, 1992:358–68.
5 McCance RA, Widdowson EM. The determinants of growth and form. *Proc R Soc Lond [B]* 1974;**185**:1–17.
6 Pauerstein CJ. *Clinical obstetrics*, chapter 20. London: Churchill Livingstone, 1987.
7 Gruenwald P. Pathology of the deprived fetus and its supply line. In: Elliott KM, Knight J, eds, *Size at birth. Ciba Foundation Symposium 27*. Amsterdam: Elsevier, 1974:3–26.
8 Campbell S, Thoms A, Ultrasound measurement of the fetal head to abdominal circumference ratios in the assessment of growth retardation. *Br J Obstet Gynaecol* 1977;**84**:165–74.
9 Carr BR, Simpson ER. Cholesterol synthesis in human fetal tissues. *J Clin Endocrinol Metab* 1982;**55**:447–52.
10 McNamara DJ, Quackenbush FW, Rodwell VW. Regulation of hepatic 3-hydroxy-3-methylglutamyl Co A reductase. *J Biol Chem* 1972;**247**:5805–10.
11 Andersen GE, Lifschitz C, Friis-Hansen B. Dietary habits and serum lipids during first 4 years of life. A study of 95 Danish children. *Acta Paediatr Scand* 1979;**68**:165–70.
12 Labarthe D, Eissa M, Vara C. Childhood precursors of high blood pressure and elevated cholesterol. *Annu Rev Public Health* 1991;**12**:519–41.
13 Sporik R, Johnstone JH, Cogswell JJ. Longitudinal study of cholesterol values in 68 children from birth to 11 years of age. *Arch Dis Child* 1991;**66**:134–7.
14 International Collaborative Study Group. Metabolic epidemiology of plasma cholesterol. Mechanism of variation of plasma cholesterol within populations and between populations. *Lancet* 1986;**ii**:991–6.
15 Fall CHD, Barker DJP, Osmond C, Winter PD, Clark PMS, Hales CN. Relation of infant feeding to adult serum cholesterol concentration and death from ischaemic heart disease. *BMJ* 1992;**304**:801–5.
16 Osmond C, Barker DJP, Winter PD, Fall CHD, Simmonds SJ. Early growth and death from cardiovascular disease in women. *BMJ* 1993;**307**:1519–24.
17 Burnside EM. Annual report of the Lady Inspector of Midwives. In: *The County Medical Officer of Health's Annual Report*. Hertfordshire, 1915.
18 Breast feeding and weaning. In: Series II: Baby. Ten minute talks to centre mothers prepared for the use of health visitors. Women Public Health Officers' Association. London, 1942:1–5.
19 Whitehead R, Paul A. Changes in infant feeding in Britain during the last century. In: *Infant feeding and cardiovascular disease: Medical Research Council Environmental Epidemiology Unit Scientific Report No. 8*. Southampton, 1987:1–10.
20 Koldovsky O, Thornburg W. Hormones in milk: A review. *J Pediatr Gastroenterol Nutr* 1987;**6**:172–96.
21 Salter AM, Fisher SC, Brindley DN. Interactions of triiodothyronine, insulin and dexamethasone on the binding of human LDL to rat hepatocytes in monolayer culture. *Atherosclerosis* 1988;**71**:77–80.
22 Lewis DS, McMahon CA, Mott GE. Breast feeding and formula feeding affect differently plasma thyroid hormone concentrations in infant baboons. *Biol Neonate* 1993;**68**:327–35.
23 Phillips DIW, Barker DJP, Osmond C. Infant feeding, fetal growth and adult thyroid function. *Acta Endocrinol* 1993;**129**:134–8.
24 Whitehead RG, Paul AA, Ahmed EA. Weaning practices in the U.K. and variations in anthropometric development. *Acta Paediatr Scand Suppl* 1986;**323**:14–25.
25 Saarinen UM. Need for iron supplementation in infants on prolonged breast feeding. *J Pediatr* 1978;**93**:177–80.

26 Belton NR. Rickets—not only the 'English Disease'. *Acta Paediatr Scand Suppl* 1986; **323**:68–75.

27 Paterson D. The next best thing: correct artificial feeding. In: *A chance for every child, A report of lectures given at the 9th Winter school for health visitors and school nurses held at Bedford College for Women, University of London Dec 30th 1929 to Jan 10th 1930.* Women Sanitary Inspectors' and Health Visitors' Association, London, 1930:22–6.

28 Kolacek S, Kapetanovic T, Zimolo A, Luzar V. Early determinants of cardiovascular risk factors in adults. A. Plasma lipids. *Acta Paediatr* 1993;**82**:699–704.

29 Morris JN. Recent history of coronary disease. *Lancet* 1951;**i**:1–7, 69–73.

30 DeWood MA, Spores J, Notske R, *et al*. Prevalence of total coronary occlusion during the early hours of transmural myocardial infarction. *N Engl J Med* 1980;**303**: 897–902.

31 Davies MJ, Thomas A. Thrombosis and acute coronary artery lesions in sudden cardiac ischemic death. *N Engl J Med* 1984;**310**:1137–40.

32 Meade TW, North WRS, Chakrabarti R, *et al*. Haemostatic function and cardiovascular death: early results of a prospective study. *Lancet* 1980;**i**:1050–4.

33 Meade TW, Mellows S, Brozovic M, *et al*. Haemostatic function and ischaemic heart disease: principal results of the Northwick Park Heart Study. *Lancet* 1986;**ii**:533–7.

34 Meade TW. The epidemiology of haemostatic and other variables in coronary artery disease. In: Verstraete M, Vermylen J, Lijnen R, Arnout J, eds, *Thrombosis and haemostasis*. Leuven, Netherlands: Leuven University Press, 1987:37–66.

35 Wilhelmsen L, Svardsudd K, Korsan-Bengtsen K, Larsson B, Welin L, Tibblin G. Fibrinogen as a risk factor for stroke and myocardial infarction. *N Engl J Med* 1984; **311**:501–5.

36 Kannel WB, Wolf PA, Castelli WP, D'Agostino RB. Fibrinogen and risk of cardiovascular disease. *JAMA* 1987;**258**:1183–6.

37 Yarnell JWG, Baker IA, Sweetnam PM, *et al*. Fibrinogen, viscosity, and white blood cell count are major risk factors for ischemic heart disease. *Circulation* 1991;**83**:836–44.

38 Ernst E, Resch KL. Fibrinogen as a cardiovascular risk factor: a meta-analysis and review of the literature. *Ann Intern Med* 1993;**118**:956–63.

39 Brozovic M. Physiological mechanisms in coagulation and fibrinolysis. *Br Med Bull* 1977;**33**:231–8.

40 Miller GJ, Martin JC, Webster J, *et al*. Association between dietary fat intake and plasma factor VII coagulant activity—a predictor of cardiovascular mortality. *Atherosclerosis* 1986;**60**:269–77.

41 Miller GJ, Cruickshank JK, Ellis LJ, *et al*. Fat consumption and factor VII coagulant activity in middle-aged men. An association between a dietary and thrombogenic coronary risk factor. *Atherosclerosis* 1989;**78**:19–24.

42 Barker DJP, Meade TW, Fall CHD, *et al*. Relation of fetal and infant growth to plasma fibrinogen and factor VII concentrations in adult life. *BMJ* 1992;**304**:148–52.

43 Andrew M, Paes B, Johnston M. Development of the hemostatic system in the neonate and young infant. *Am J Pediatr Hematol Oncol* 1990;**12**:95–104.

44 Holmes GE, Miller HC, Hassanein K, Lanksy SB, Goggin JE. Postnatal somatic growth in infants with atypical fetal growth patterns. *Am J Dis Child* 1977;**131**: 1078–83.

45 Villar J, Smeriglio V, Martorell R, Brown CH, Klein RE. Heterogeneous growth and mental development of intrauterine growth retarded infants during the first 3 years of life. *Pediatrics* 1984;**74**:783–91.

46 Marmot MG, Shipley MJ, Rose G. Inequalities in death—specific explanations of a general pattern? *Lancet* 1984;**i**:1003–6.

47 Waaler HT. Height, weight and mortality. The Norwegian experience. *Acta Med Scand [Suppl]* 1984;**679**:1–56.

48 Notkola V. *Living conditions in childhood and coronary heart disease in adulthood*. Helsinki: Finnish Society of Sciences and Letters, 1985.

6: Non-insulin dependent diabetes

Non-insulin dependent diabetes increases the risk of coronary heart disease and is associated with hypertension.[1][2] Insulin has a central role in fetal growth, and disorders of glucose and insulin metabolism are therefore a possible link between early growth and cardiovascular disease.[3] Although obesity and a sedentary lifestyle are known to be important in the development of non-insulin dependent diabetes, they seem to lead to the disease only in predisposed individuals. Family and twin studies have suggested that the predisposition is familial, but the search for genetic markers has been unrewarding. This chapter describes studies of the relationship between fetal growth and diabetes which have led to a new explanation of the origins of the disease, the so called "thrifty phenotype" hypothesis.

Table 6.1 shows the results of a study by Hales and colleagues[4] in which 370 men in Hertfordshire were given a standard oral glucose challenge. Plasma glucose concentrations obtained two hours after ingestion of glucose were used to identify men with diabetes (plasma glucose $\geqslant 11\cdot1$ mmol/l) or the precursor disorder, impaired glucose tolerance (plasma glucose $7\cdot8–11\cdot0$ mmol/l). The proportion of men with either disorder fell pro-

TABLE 6.1—*Percentages of men aged 64 years with impaired glucose tolerance (two hour glucose $7\cdot8–11\cdot0$ mmol/l) or diabetes (two hour glucose $\geqslant 11\cdot1$ mmol/l) according to birthweight*

| Birthweight (lb)* | Number of men | Percentage of men with two hour glucose of: | | | Odds ratio adjusted for body mass index (95% confidence interval) |
		$7\cdot8–11\cdot0$ mmol/l	$\geqslant 11\cdot1$ mmol/l	$\geqslant 7\cdot8$ mmol/l	
$\leqslant 5\cdot5$	20	30	10	40	6·6 (1·5–28)
−6·5	47	21	13	34	4·8 (1·3–17)
−7·5	104	25	6	31	4·6 (1·4–16)
−8·5	117	15	7	22	2·6 (0·8–8·9)
−9·5	54	4	9	13	1·4 (0·3–5·6)
>9·5	28	14	0	14	1·0 —
All	370	18	7	25	*p* value for trend <0·001

*1 lb = 454 g.

TABLE 6.2—*Percentages of men aged 64 years with impaired glucose tolerance (two hour glucose 7·8–11·0 mmol/l) or diabetes (two hour glucose ≥ 11·1 mmol/l) according to weight at one year*

Weight at 1 year (lb)*	Number of men	Percentage of men with two hour glucose of			Odds ratio adjusted for body mass index (95% confidence interval)
		7·8–11·0 mmol/l	≥ 11·1 mmol/l	≥ 7·8 mmol/l	
≤ 18	23	26	17	43	8·2 (1·8–38)
−20	63	21	11	32	4·8 (1·2–19)
−22	107	22	7	30	4·2 (1·1–16)
−24	105	13	5	18	2·1 (0·5–7·9)
−26	48	13	6	19	2·1 (0·5–9·0)
≥ 27	24	13	0	13	1·0 —
All	370	18	7	25	*p* value for trend <0·001

*1 lb = 454 g.

TABLE 6.3—*Mean plasma glucose two hours after 75 g oral glucose load, according to weight at one year and adult body mass index in men aged 64 years*

Adult body mass index (kg/m²)	Weight at one year in lb (kg)			
	≤ 21·5 (≤ 9·75)	−23·5 (−10·66)	>23·5 (>10·66)	All
≤ 25·4	6·6 (45)	6·1 (39)	5·8 (36)	6·2 (120)
−28	6·7 (47)	6·9 (44)	5·9 (36)	6·5 (127)
>28	7·7 (39)	7·4 (43)	6·6 (41)	7·2 (123)
All	7·0 (131)	6·8 (126)	6·1 (113)	6·6 (370)

Numbers of men in parentheses.

gressively from those with the lowest to those with the highest birthweights. The differences in prevalence were threefold and the differences in relative risk, taking account of current body mass, were sevenfold. Trends with weight at one year of age were similar to those seen with birthweight (table 6.2). Fasting plasma glucose concentrations were not related to early weight, but 30 minute plasma glucose and two hour plasma glucose and insulin concentrations fell sharply from men with low birthweight and weight at one year of age to those who were larger. In each social class and at each level of body mass, there was the same relationship between low weight gain *in utero* and during infancy, and impaired glucose tolerance 60 years later.

Table 6.3 shows the plasma glucose concentrations at two hours with the men divided into approximate thirds according to weight at one year of age and adult body mass index. The values rise from 5·8 mmol/l in men with the highest weights at one year of age and lowest body mass indices to 7·7 mmol/l in men with the lowest weights at one year of age and highest body mass indices. Fetal and infant growth therefore protect against the deleterious effect of higher body mass in adult life and, conversely, lower body mass protects against the deleterious effect of reduced early growth. Forty one per cent of men whose birthweight and weight at one year of age were below the median, and whose body mass indices were above the median, had impaired glucose tolerance or diabetes. Only 6% of men who were above the median for early weights and below the median for body mass index were affected.

In the Hertfordshire study the only recorded measurement of body size at birth was birthweight; the study was therefore repeated among the men and women in Preston (page 54). Of the 393 people who lived in or close to Preston, 266 agreed to undergo a standard oral glucose tolerance test.[5] Of these 34 had impaired glucose tolerance or newly diagnosed diabetes, and the prevalence of these disorders fell progressively from 27% in those with birthweight of 5·5 lb or less ($\leqslant$2·5 kg) to 6% in those with birthweight 7·5 lb or more ($\geqslant$3·4 kg). After allowing for differences in current body mass, the relative risk fell from 6·4 to 1·0. As in the Hertfordshire study, plasma glucose concentrations at 30 minutes and two hours fell with increasing birthweight, and there were corresponding trends in two hour insulin concentrations. These trends were barely changed by adjustments for duration of gestation, and therefore reflected differences in fetal growth rates.

In the Hertfordshire and Preston studies, two hour plasma glucose concentrations fell progressively up to the highest birthweights so that people with birthweights of more than 9·5 lb (>4·31 kg) had the lowest concentrations. As mothers with diabetes in pregnancy tend to have large babies one might expect some large babies to show evidence of impaired glucose metabolism. This effect may not be apparent in those two studies because the number of such babies is small in relation to the number of babies who are heavy because of good fetal nutrition. In a study of Pima Indians, however, young men and women with birthweights over 9·9 lb (>4·5 kg) had an increased prevalence of non-insulin dependent diabetes as did those with birthweights below 5·5 lb (<2·5 kg).[6] The increased risk of diabetes among babies with high birthweights was associated with maternal diabetes in pregnancy, which is unusually common in Pima Indians.

The Preston study showed that both thin (see fig 3.8) and short babies (see fig 3.9) tend to develop impaired glucose tolerance and diabetes. These associations are being examined further in Sheffield, where low birthweight is again strongly linked to impaired glucose tolerance (unpublished data). People in Preston with impaired glucose tolerance had an increased placental weight: birthweight ratio, suggesting that diabetes is linked to fetal undernutrition.

The mechanisms linking low fetal and infant growth rates with adult glucose intolerance are not known. There is evidence, however, that both insulin deficiency caused by pancreatic β cell dysfunction and insulin resistance may be determined in fetal life. Both deficiency and resistance are thought to be important in the pathogenesis of non-insulin dependent diabetes.[7]

Insulin deficiency

Much of the development of the islets of Langerhans occurs *in utero*.[8] The exact timing of islet formation differs among species. In rats the number of islets increases rapidly in the last 4–6 days of intrauterine life. In humans β cell mass increases more than 130-fold between the twelfth intrauterine week and the fifth postnatal month. There are few studies of the effects on β cell development of undernutrition during early life. Studies in animals show that undernutrition *in utero* or during early postnatal life may reduce the number of β cells and the secretion of insulin[9–11] (see p. 26). In rats weaned on a low protein diet for only three weeks, the insulin response to glucose was permanently impaired, leading to the suggestion "that early malnutrition may predispose to diabetes".[10] Infants who are small for dates have fewer β cells.[8] There are conflicting reports on whether the β cell mass is reduced in patients with non-insulin dependent diabetes.[12] In one study, however, in which diabetic patients were compared with people of the same weight, their β cell mass was found to be lower.[13] As a working hypothesis it seems reasonable to propose that nutritional and other factors determining fetal and infant growth influence the size and function of the adult pancreatic β cell complement. Whether and when non-insulin dependent diabetes supervenes will be determined by the rate of attrition of β cells with ageing, and by the development of insulin resistance, of which obesity is an important determinant.

Recent advances in assay methodology make it possible to measure specifically plasma concentrations of the precursor of insulin—32–33 split proinsulin.[14 15] A raised plasma split proinsulin concentration is thought to indicate β cell dysfunction. Table 6.4 shows the plasma concentrations of this split proinsulin among men in the Hertfordshire study, divided into approximate thirds according to weight at one year of age and adult body mass index, as in table 6.3.[4] The values rise from 2·1 pmol/l in men with the highest weights at one year of age and lowest body mass indices to 4·8 pmol/l in men with the lowest weight at one year of age and highest body mass indices. These findings are consistent with the hypothesis that

TABLE 6.4—*Geometric mean plasma 32–33 split proinsulin concentrations (pmol/l) according to weight at one year and adult body mass index in men aged 64 years*

Adult body mass index (kg/m²)	Weight at one year in lb (kg)			
	≤21·5 (≤9·75)	−23·5 (−10·66)	>23·5 (>10·66)	All
≤25·4	2·5 (57)	2·2 (56)	2·1 (49)	2·2 (162)
−28	3·2 (57)	3·6 (49)	3·1 (41)	3·3 (147)
>28	4·8 (48)	3·8 (59)	3·9 (52)	4·1 (159)
All	3·3 (162)	3·1 (164)	2·9 (142)	3·1 (468)

Numbers of men in parentheses.

the relationship between low birthweight and diabetes depends partly on impaired development of the endocrine pancreas.

In a sample of 103 of the men and women who took part in the Preston study, Phillips and colleagues[16] measured insulin secretion following intravenous infusion of glucose. The insulin response was not related to birthweight or other measurements at birth. This argues against a link between reduced fetal growth and insulin deficiency in adult life. It is possible that insulin resistance in adult life changes insulin secretion and obscures associations with fetal growth. Studies of younger people may resolve this—a study of young men aged 21 years by Robinson and colleagues[17] showed that those with lower birthweight had reduced plasma insulin concentrations at 30 minutes.

Insulin resistance

Whereas the association of reduced fetal growth with insulin deficiency is uncertain, that with insulin resistance is becoming increasingly clear. Men and women with low birthweight have a high prevalence of the "insulin resistance syndrome", syndrome X, in which impaired glucose tolerance, hypertension, and raised serum triglyceride concentrations occur in the same patient. The patients are insulin resistant and have hyperinsulinaemia. Table 6.5 shows results for a sample of the men in the Hertfordshire study. The prevalence of the syndrome falls progressively from 30% in men who weighed 5·5 lb or less (≤2·5 kg) at birth to 6% in those who weighed 9·5 lb or more (≥4·3 kg).[18] A study in Preston gave similar results, and showed a similar relationship in men and women. The association with low birth-weight was independent of the duration of gestation and therefore depended on low rates of fetal growth.

A recent study in San Antonio, Texas, confirmed the association in a different ethnic group. In 30-year-old Mexican–Americans and non-His-

TABLE 6.5—*Prevalence of syndrome X (type 2 diabetes, hypertension, and hyperlipidaemia) in men aged 64 years, according to birthweight*

Birthweight (lb)*	Total number of men	Percentage with syndrome X	Odds ratio adjusted for body mass index (95% confidence interval)
≤5·5	20	30	18 (2·6–118)
−6·5	54	19	8·4 (1·5–49)
−7·5	114	17	8·5 (1·5–46)
−8·5	123	12	4·9 (0·9–27)
−9·5	64	6	2·2 (0·3–14)
>9·5	32	6	1·0
Total	407	14	p value for trend <0·001

*1 lb = 454 g.

panic white people, those with lower birthweight had a higher prevalence of the insulin resistance syndrome.[19] Among men and women in the lowest third of the birthweight distribution and the highest third of current body mass 25% had the syndrome. By contrast none of the people in the highest third of birthweight and lowest third of current body mass had it.

These findings point to a link between impaired fetal growth and insulin resistance in later life. This possibility is encouraged by the observation in Hertfordshire that low birthweight is linked to a tendency to store fat abdominally in later life, known to be a marker of insulin resistance.[20] In San Antonio low birthweight was not associated with abdominal fat deposition, as measured by a high waist : hip ratio, but rather was associated with fat storage on the trunk, as measured by a high subscapular : triceps skinfold thickness ratio.[19] Phillips and colleagues[21] carried out insulin tolerance tests on 103 men and women in Preston. Table 6.6 shows the findings, with insulin resistance expressed as the time taken for the plasma glucose concentration to fall to half its initial value after intravenous injection of insulin. The men and women are subdivided according to ponderal index at birth and current body mass index. At each body mass, resistance was greater in those with a low ponderal index. Conversely, at each ponderal index, resistance was greater in those with high body mass, and the greatest mean resistance was therefore in those with low ponderal index at birth but high current body mass.

The processes that link thinness at birth with insulin resistance in adult life are not known. Studies of patients with non-insulin dependent diabetes, using a euglycaemic clamp, have shown that peripheral tissues, particularly skeletal muscle, are an important site of insulin resistance.[7] Muscle biopsies have shown that insulin resistance is associated with a lower density of capillaries in muscle, a lesser proportion of type 1 muscle fibres, and a greater proportion of type 2B fibres.[22] Transcapillary insulin transport is a rate limiting step in insulin action.[23] Babies born at term with a low ponderal

TABLE 6.6—*Mean insulin resistance (half life of blood glucose in minutes) in men and women aged 50 years according to ponderal index at birth and adult body mass*

Ponderal index at birth (kg/m³)	Body mass index (kg/m²)				
	≤24·0	−26·0	−28·0	>28·0	All
≤20·6	17·9 (8)	18·0 (8)	23·1 (4)	30·7 (6)	20·6 (26)
−22·3	15·8 (16)	17·3 (11)	17·8 (6)	27·1 (4)	17·3 (37)
−25·0	14·4 (8)	20·7 (4)	21·0 (3)	20·4 (8)	17·9 (23)
>25·0	14·1 (4)	16·1 (4)	17·8 (3)	18·5 (6)	16·6 (17)
All	15·6 (36)	17·7 (27)	19·5 (16)	22·6 (24)	18·0 (103)

Figures in parentheses are number of people.

index have a reduced mid-arm circumference, which implies that they have a low muscle bulk as well as less subcutaneous fat.[24] It is therefore possible that thinness at birth is associated with abnormalities in muscle structure and function which develop in mid-gestation and persist into adult life, interfering with insulin's ability to promote glucose uptake.

Reavens[24] has suggested that non-insulin dependent diabetes, hypertension, hypertriglyceridaemia, low HDL cholesterol concentrations, and the other abnormalities of syndrome X coexist because they are all consequences of insulin resistance and hyperinsulinaemia.[25] The mechanisms by which insulin resistance could give rise to this spectrum of abnormalities are unknown. If insulin resistance is a consequence of impaired fetal development, it precedes the development of syndrome X and could therefore cause it. The weak relationship between plasma insulin concentrations and blood pressure in clinical and epidemiological studies is, however, consistent with the hypothesis that the components of syndrome X are associated because they have a common origin in suboptimal development *in utero*.[26]

Studies of children and young adults

The findings that have been described lead to the conclusion that fetal undernutrition in mid to late gestation gives rise to insulin resistance in peripheral tissues, including muscle, and impairs growth of the endocrine pancreas.

A survey of 20-year-old men in Britain, and two surveys of young Mexican–Americans and Pima Indians in the USA, demonstrated the same relationship between reduced glucose tolerance and low birthweight as

TABLE 6.7—*Mean plasma glucose concentrations at 30 minutes and mean blood pressures in seven-year-old children by ponderal index at birth*

Ponderal index (kg/m³)	Mean plasma glucose concentration (mmol/l) at 30 minutes			Mean blood pressure at four years (mm Hg)*
	Boys	Girls	Total	
≤23·0	8·35 (24)	8·64 (22)	8·49 (46)	107 (46)
−25·0	8·18 (20)	8·16 (21)	8·17 (41)	107 (40)
−27·5	8·35 (29)	8·18 (29)	8·27 (58)	105 (57)
>27·5	7·61 (28)	8·27 (33)	7·97 (61)	103 (61)
Total	8·11 (101)	8·30 (105)	8·21 (206)	105 (204)
s.d.	1·54	1·58	1·57	9
p value for trend			0·04	0·05

Numbers of children in parentheses.
*After adjustment for weight at four years.

seen in older adults.[6 17 19] This raised the question of whether the relationship could be demonstrated in children. Such a demonstration would be further evidence that the pathogenesis of non-insulin dependent diabetes is set in train in fetal life, and would show that metabolism becomes impaired within a few years of birth.

Two hundred and fifty of the children in Salisbury, England, now aged seven years, who had taken part in the study of blood pressure at the age of four years (page 56), were still living in the district and were willing to take part in a study of glucose tolerance.[27] The test was not continued beyond 30 minutes after a standard oral glucose load. Children who had been the heaviest babies had the lowest plasma glucose concentrations at 30 minutes, although there was no trend from the lowest to the highest birthweight groups. Ponderal index at birth was more strongly related to 30 minute glucose. Table 6.7 shows that 30 minute glucose concentrations were highest in boys and girls who had been thinnest at birth; it also shows the blood pressures recorded at four years of age were again highest in children who were thinnest at birth.[28]

These findings in children provide further support for the hypothesis that non-insulin dependent diabetes originates from impaired development in mid to late gestation. In addition there were interesting differences in the associations of the two insulin precursors—proinsulin and 32–33 split proinsulin—with size at birth. Plasma concentrations of both precursors rose with increasing current weight, but the split proinsulin concentrations, which were high in comparison with those found in adults, also rose with decreasing length at birth. One possibility is that this association reflects the effects of fetal undernutrition in late gestation, with consequent reduction in linear growth and failure of pancreatic development.

87

TABLE 6.8—*Mean 30 minute plasma glucose and insulin concentrations among four-year-old children in India*

Birthweight (kg)	Plasma glucose at 30 min (mmol/l)	Plasma insulin at 30 min (pmol/l)	Number of children
≤2·4	8·14	334	36
–2·6	8·26	330	36
–2·8	7·74	293	44
–3·0	7·81	288	42
>3·0	7·39	262	43
All	7·84	299	201
p value for trend	0·01*	0·04†	

*Allowing for the children's current weight.
†Allowing for the children's age, sex, and current weight.

The findings in the Salisbury study are echoed by similar findings made by Yajnik and colleagues in four-year-old children in Pune, India (unpublished data). The distribution of their birthweights, shown in table 6.8, reflects the low mean birthweight which prevails in India.[29] The 30 minute plasma glucose and insulin concentrations fell from children with the lowest to those with the highest birthweight. The high insulin concentrations of children who were small at birth are consistent with the hypothesis that growth failure *in utero* leads to resistance to insulin. Insulin resistance is known to be common in adult Indians, and is linked to the unusually high prevalence of non-insulin dependent diabetes in India.[30] As in the Salisbury study, blood pressure also fell with increasing birthweight. Length at birth was not measured routinely and the ponderal index could not therefore be calculated.

The "thrifty phenotype" hypothesis

The associations between body size at birth and impaired glucose tolerance in adults and children led to what Hales has called the "thrifty phenotype" hypothesis.[31] The essence of the hypothesis is that poor nutrition in fetal and early infant life is detrimental to the development and function of the β cells of the islets of Langerhans, and changes the tissues, primarily muscle, which respond to insulin, and as a consequence this leads to insulin resistance. Deficiency in insulin production or in the sensitivity of tissues to it predisposes to the development of non-insulin dependent diabetes; adult influences, including obesity, ageing, and physical inactivity, determine the time of onset and severity of the disease.

According to the thrifty phenotype hypothesis, non-insulin dependent diabetes is the outcome of the undernourished fetus and infant having to be nutritionally thrifty. For as long as the individual remains under-

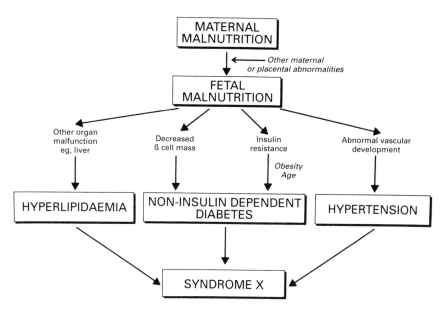

FIG 6.1—*The fetal origins of non-insulin dependent diabetes and syndrome X: the "thrifty phenotype" hypothesis.*

nourished, its glucose–insulin metabolism is adequate. A sudden move to over- or good nutrition, however, exposes the deficiencies in β cell function, and tissue sensitivity and diabetes result.

The thrifty phenotype hypothesis is shown diagrammatically in the figure which also outlines how the features of syndrome X may originate in failure of early development. The hypothesis demands a reinterpretation of some data and explains other observations which at present are not easy to understand.

Geographical variations and migrant studies

The prevalence of non-insulin dependent diabetes varies in different countries and in different parts of the same country. Rates tend to be lower in places that have retained a traditional lifestyle, for example, rural Africa, where the prevalence in adults is between 1 and 2%, or the highlands of Papua New Guinea, where there was a complete absence of diabetes in one survey.[32][33] Prevalences in European and white North American populations are typically around 5% among adults.[34] Populations exposed to rapid Westernisation have a higher prevalence than European populations. The highest known prevalences occur in North American and western Pacific societies where up to one third of the adult population may be affected. The best studied of these are the Pima Indian and Nauruan islanders.[35][36]

The proposal that the disease is the outcome of reduced early growth is consistent with these geographical variations. If undernutrition during fetal life and infancy results in insensitivity to insulin and impaired function of the β cells of the islets of Langerhans, later overnutrition may expose the impaired function and lead to diabetes. A rapid transition from subsistence to overnutrition could explain the high diabetes rate in the Nauruan islanders. These people suffered severe nutritional deficiency before and during the Second World War. After the war they suddenly became affluent as a result of phosphate mining, and diabetes became epidemic on the island. A similar sudden transition occurred in Ethiopian Jews who were recently transported to Israel and have developed a high prevalence of diabetes.[37]

Twins and family studies

Evidence for a genetic aetiology of non-insulin dependent diabetes comes from twin studies and a study of family pedigrees. Three studies—two in the USA and one in the UK[38-40]—of twin pairs found a higher concordance rate in monozygotic twins when the age of onset of the proband was more than 40 years, that is, the diabetes was non-insulin dependent. Although two of these studies are likely to have been affected by serious ascertainment bias, the most recent study was carried out using a population based sample of twins identified from military records.[40] Twin pairs were examined twice, at a mean age of 47 years and then at 57 years. At the first examination, when the prevalence rate was 5·7%, there was no difference in concordance rates between monozygotic and dizygotic twins. Ten years later, however, the disease prevalence rate was 13% and the concordance rate, in monozygotic twins, 58·3%, compared with 17·4% in dizygotic twins.

In a large study in Canada of 3117 patients with non-insulin dependent diabetes, the risk of the disease was increased between two- and fourfold in the siblings of probands with the disease.[41] Similar findings were observed in the Whitehall surveys of civil servants.[42] In populations with a higher prevalence of glucose intolerance, familial clustering of the disease is more marked. Thus in the Nauruan islanders, glucose intolerance develops in approximately 40% of the offspring of two diabetic parents, in 6% of offspring if one parent is diabetic, and in none of the children if the parents have normal glucose tolerance.[43]

The observations of familial clustering of diabetes, a high concordance rate in monozygotic twins, and the high prevalence rate in communities that have abandoned their traditional lifestyle and adopted a Western diet led Neel to suggest the "thrifty genotype" hypothesis.[44] He proposed that genes existed which gave a survival advantage in harsh conditions when food was scarce. In times of plenty, however, the same genes were detrimental, leading to obesity and glucose intolerance.

The evidence presented here raises a question about the interpretation of family and twin data as evidence for genetic inheritance. As maternal physique and nutrition have such a strong influence on fetal and infant growth (see chapter 9), the reason for the familial clustering of diabetes may be that family members share a similar early environment. A stronger maternal than paternal influence on the development of diabetes is consistent with this hypothesis.[45] Likewise, a genetic interpretation of high concordance rates in monozygotic twins may not be justifiable because identical twins share a common early environment, in particular a common placenta.[46]

Summary

Five studies have shown that men and women who had low birthweight have increased rates of non-insulin dependent diabetes, and impaired glucose tolerance. People who were thin at birth, having a low muscle bulk, tend to become insulin resistant and develop syndrome X—diabetes, hypertension, and raised plasma triglycerides. These abnormalities may have a common origin in suboptimal development at a particular stage of gestation.

The "thrifty phenotype" hypothesis offers an explanation of the epidemiology of non-insulin dependent diabetes. The hypothesis proposes that poor nutrition in fetal and early infant life is detrimental to the mechanisms maintaining carbohydrate tolerance. It may affect the structure and function of the β cells of the islets of Langerhans, and may change the tissues, primarily muscle, which respond to insulin and as a consequence lead to insulin resistance. Although these early changes determine susceptibility to non-insulin dependent diabetes, additional factors such as obesity, ageing, and physical inactivity must also play a part in determining the time of onset and severity of the disease.

1 Fuller JH, Shipley MJ, Rose G, Jarrett RJ, Keen H. Coronary heart disease risk and impaired glucose tolerance. *Lancet* 1980;**i**:1373–6.
2 Modan M, Halkin H, Almog S, *et al.* Hyperinsulinaemia: a link between hypertension, obesity and glucose intolerance. *J Clin Invest* 1985;**75**:809–17.
3 Fowden AL. The role of insulin in prenatal growth. *J Dev Physiol* 1989;**12**:173–82.
4 Hales CN, Barker DJP, Clark PMS, *et al.* Fetal and infant growth and impaired glucose tolerance at age 64. *BMJ* 1991;**303**:1019–22.
5 Phipps K, Barker DJP, Hales CN, Fall CHD, Osmond C, Clark PMS. Fetal growth and impaired glucose tolerance in men and women. *Diabetologia* 1993;**36**:225–8.

6 McCance DR, Pettit DJ, Hanson RL, Jacobsson LTM, Knowle WC, Bennett PH. Birthweight and non-insulin dependent diabetes: "thrifty genotype", "thrifty phenotype", or "surviving small baby genotype". *BMJ* 1994;**308**:942–5.

7 DeFronzo RA. The triumvirate: beta cell, muscle, liver. A collusion responsible for NIDDM. *Diabetes* 1988;**37**:667–87.

8 Van Assche FA, Aerts L. The fetal endocrine pancreas. *Contrib Gynecol Obstet* 1979;**5**: 44–57.

9 Weinkove C, Weinkove EA, Pimstone BL. Insulin release and pancreatic islet volume in malnourished rats. *S Afr Med J* 1974;**48**:1888.

10 Swenne I, Crace CJ, Milner RDG. Persistent impairment of insulin secretory response to glucose in adult rats after limited periods of protein-calorie malnutrition early in life. *Diabetes* 1987;**36**:454–8.

11 Snoeck A, Remacle C, Reusens B, Hoet JJ. Effect of a low protein diet during pregnancy on the fetal rat endocrine pancreas. *Biol Neonate* 1990;**5**:107–18.

12 Hellerström C, Swenne I, Andersson A. Islet cell replication and diabetes. In: Lefebvre PJ, Pipeleers DG, eds, *The pathology of the endocrine pancreas in diabetes*. Heidelberg: Springer Verlag, 1988:141–70.

13 Klöppel G, Löhr M, Habich K, Oberholzer M, Heitz PU. Islet pathology and pathogenesis of type 1 and type 2 diabetes mellitus revisited. *Survey and Synthesis of Pathology Research* 1985;**4**:110–25.

14 Sobey WJ, Beer SF, Carrington CA, *et al*. Sensitive and specific two-site immunoradiometric assays for human insulin, proinsulin, 65–66 split and 32–33 split proinsulins. *Biochem J* 1989;**260**:535–41.

15 Temple RC, Carrington CA, Luzio SD, *et al*. Insulin deficiency in non-insulin dependent diabetes. *Lancet* 1989;**i**:294–5.

16 Phillips DIW, Hirst S, Clark PMS, Hales CN, Osmond C. Fetal growth and insulin secretion in adult life. *Diabetologia* 1994;**37**:(in press).

17 Robinson S, Walton RJ, Clark PM, Barker DJP, Hales CN, Osmond C. The relation of fetal growth to plasma glucose in young men. *Diabetologia* 1992;**35**:444–6.

18 Barker DJP, Hales CN, Fall CHD, Osmond C, Phipps K, Clark PMS. Type 2 (non-insulin-dependent) diabetes mellitus, hypertension and hyperlipidaemia (syndrome X): relation to reduced fetal growth. *Diabetologia* 1993;**36**:62–7.

19 Valdez R, Athens MA, Thompson GH, Bradshaw BS, Stern MP. Birthweight and adult health outcomes in a biethnic population in the USA. *Diabetologia* 1994;**37**:624–31.

20 Law CM, Barker DJP, Osmond C, Fall CHD, Simmonds SJ. Early growth and abdominal fatness in adult life. *J Epidemiol Community Health* 1992;**46**:184–6.

21 Phillips DIW, Barker DJP, Hales CN, Hirst S, Osmond C. Thinness at birth and insulin resistance in adult life. *Diabetologia* 1994;**37**:150–4.

22 Lillioja S, Young AA, Cutler CL, *et al*. Skeletal muscle capillary density and fiber type are possible determinants of in vivo insulin resistance in man. *J Clin Invest* 1987;**80**: 415–24.

23 Bergman RN, Yang YJ, Hope ID, Ader M. The role of the transcapillary insulin transport in the efficiency of insulin action: studies with glucose clamps and the minimal model. *Horm Metab Res Suppl* 1990;**24**:49–56.

24 Robinson SM, Wheeler T, Hayes MC, Barker DJP, Osmond C. Fetal heart rate and intrauterine growth. *Br J Obstet Gynaecol* 1991;**98**:1223–7.

25 Reaven GM. Banting lecture 1988. Role of insulin resistance in human disease. *Diabetes* 1988;**37**:1595–607.

26 Jarrett RJ. In defence of insulin: a critique of syndrome X. *Lancet* 1992;**340**:469–71.

27 Law CM, Gordon GS, Shiell AW, Barker DJP, Hales CN. Thinness at birth and glucose tolerance in seven year old children. *Diabetic Medicine* (in press).

28 Law CM, Barker DJP, Bull AR, Osmond C. Maternal and fetal influences on blood pressure. *Arch Dis Child* 1991;**66**:1291–5.

29 Mohan M, Shiv Prasad SR, Chellani HK, Kapani V. Intrauterine growth curves in North Indian babies: weight, length, head circumference and ponderal index. *Indian Paediatrics* 1990;**27**:43–51.

30 Ramachandran A. Epidemiology of diabetes in Indians. *Int J Diab Dev Countries* 1993; **13**:65–7.

31 Hales CN, Barker DJP. Type 2 (non-insulin-dependent) diabetes mellitus: the thrifty phenotype hypothesis. *Diabetologia* 1992;**35**:595–601.

32 McLarty DG, Kintange HM, Mtinangi BL, *et al*. Prevalence of diabetes and impaired glucose tolerance in rural Tanzania. *Lancet* 1989;**i**:871–4.

33 King H, Heywood P, Zimmet P, *et al*. Glucose tolerance in a highland population in Papua New Guinea. *Diabetes Res* 1984;**1**:45–51.

34 Butler WJ, Ostrander LD Jr, Carman WJ, *et al*. Diabetes mellitus in Tecumseh, Michigan: prevalence, incidence, and associated conditions. *Am J Epidemiol* 1982; **116**:971–80.

35 Knowle WC, Bennett PH, Hamman RF, Miller M. Diabetes incidence in the Pima Indians: a 19-fold greater incidence than in Rochester, Minnesota. *Am J Epidemiol* 1978;**108**:497–504.

36 Zimmet P, King H, Taylor R, *et al*. The high prevalence of diabetes mellitus, impaired glucose tolerance and diabetic retinopathy in Nauru: the 1982 survey. *Diabetes Res* 1984;**1**:13–18.

37 Cohen MP, Stern E, Rusecki Y, Zeidler A. High prevalence of diabetes in young adult Ethiopian immigrants to Israel. *Diabetes* 1988;**37**:824–8.

38 Gottlieb MS, Root HF. Diabetes mellitus in twins. *Diabetes* 1968;**17**:693–704.

39 Barnett AH, Eff C, Leslie RDG, Pyke DA. Diabetes in identical twins: a study of 200 pairs. *Diabetologia* 1981;**20**:87–93.

40 Newman B, Selby JV, King MC, *et al*. Concordance for type 2 (non-insulin dependent) diabetes mellitus in male twins. *Diabetologia* 1987;**30**:763–8.

41 Simpson NR. Diabetes in the families of diabetics. *Can Med Assoc J* 1968;**98**:427–32.

42 Keen H, Jarrett RJ. Environmental factors and genetic interactions. In: Creutzfeldt W, Köbberling J, Neel JV, eds, *The genetics of diabetes mellitus*. Berlin: Springer-Verlag, 1976:115–24.

43 Serjeantson SW, Zimmet P. Diabetes in the Pacific: evidence for a major gene. In: Baba S, Gould M, Zimmet P, eds, *Diabetes mellitus: recent knowledge on aetiology, complications and treatment*. Sydney: Academic Press, 1984:23–30.

44 Neel JV. Diabetes mellitus: a 'thrifty' genotype rendered detrimental by 'progress'? *Am J Hum Gen* 1962;**14**:353–62.

45 Alcolado JC, Alcolado R. Importance of maternal history of non-insulin dependent diabetic patients. *BMJ* 1991;**302**:1178–80.

46 Phillips DIW. Twin studies in medical research: can they tell us whether diseases are genetically determined? *Lancet* 1993;**341**:1008–9.

7: Chronic bronchitis

For many years there has been interest in the hypothesis that lower respiratory tract infection during infancy and early childhood causes chronic bronchitis in later life.[1-6] (In this chapter the term "chronic bronchitis" is used instead of the more precise, but less familiar, "chronic airflow obstruction".) The broad similarity in the international geography and time trends of respiratory disease at different ages was an early pointer to this.[3] Migrant studies also suggested that determinants of chronic bronchitis act in early life. Among British born men who migrated to the USA, the prevalence of chronic bronchitis was higher than among migrants from Norway.[7] The differences persisted after allowing for smoking habits and were unrelated to the men's age at migration. The prevalence was also higher among men born in urban rather than rural areas of Britain. It was later shown that people born in cities and large towns in Britain have an increased risk of death from chronic bronchitis irrespective of where they move to, either within or outside the country.[7 8]

Until recently there was little direct evidence that respiratory infection in early life had long term effects. Bronchiolitis, bronchitis, and pneumonia in infancy were shown to be followed by persisting damage to the airways during childhood, with cough, wheeze, bronchial reactivity, and impaired ventilatory function;[9-12] and in the long term follow up of a national sample of 3899 British children born in 1946, young adults who had had one or more lower respiratory infections before two years of age were found to have a higher prevalence of chronic cough.[13-15] Recently, however, a geographical study and two follow up studies of men born 60 or more years ago have added to the evidence.

Geography

Death rates from chronic bronchitis vary widely among different places in England and Wales. Fig 7.1 shows rates among men in each of the 1366 local authority areas during 1968-78:[16] rates are highest in the cities and large towns, and lowest in the rural areas. The distributions are similar in men and women, although rates in women are much lower—269 deaths per million per year compared with 848 in men. Detailed studies of death certificates and the findings of prevalence surveys in Britain show that geographical differences in mortality certified as caused by chronic bronchitis

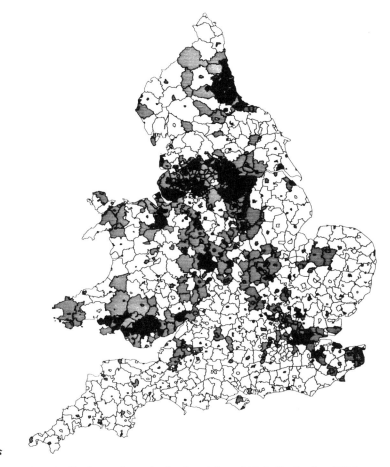

FIG 7.1—*Standardised mortality ratios for chronic bronchitis in England and Wales among men aged 35–74 years.* ■ = *High*; ▦ = *medium*; □ = *low.*

and emphysema reflect differences in the prevalence of these diseases.[17] In figs 7.2 and 7.3 the death rates among men and women are compared with infant deaths from bronchitis and pneumonia during 1921–25, the earliest period for which such data are available. In the same way as in the geographical studies of cardiovascular disease (see chapter 1), the local authority areas are grouped into 212 areas, comprising large towns, London boroughs, all small towns within each county, and all rural areas within each county. The distribution of adult deaths from chronic bronchitis correlates remarkably strongly with past infant deaths, the correlation coefficients being 0·84 in men (fig 7.2) and 0·80 in women (fig 7.3). The correlations are also specific. Past infant death rates from bronchitis and

95

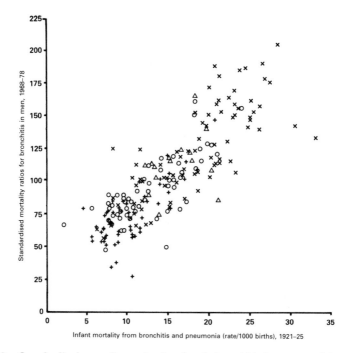

FIG 7.2—*Standardised mortality ratios for chronic bronchitis in men aged 35–74, and past infant mortality rates from bronchitis and pneumonia in England and Wales.*

pneumonia correlate more closely with current adult death rates from chronic bronchitis than with any other cause of death, current or past, adult or infant.

Most deaths from chronic bronchitis occurring at age 35–74 years during 1968–78 occurred among people born before 1921–25, the earliest years for which cause specific infant mortality data were published. Total postneonatal death rates are, however, available from 1911 and may be used as a proxy for respiratory deaths in infants, because respiratory infection was the main cause of postneonatal mortality.[18] The correlation coefficients between postneonatal mortality and adult mortality from bronchitis during 1968–78, in both sexes, were the same ($r = 0.83$) for postneonatal rates throughout 1911–20 as for 1921–25.

It could be argued that the similar geographical distribution of infant deaths from respiratory infection and adult deaths from bronchitis simply reflects persistence over the years of geograhical differences in environmental influences which determine respiratory disease at all ages. Air temperature is an example of such an influence.[19] Several determinants of chronic bronchitis, however, act only at certain ages.[20] The risk of infant respiratory

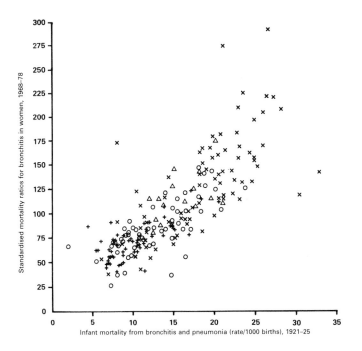

FIG 7.3—*Standardised mortality ratios for chronic bronchitis in women aged 35–74, and past infant mortality rates from bronchitis and pneumonia in England and Wales.*

infection is reduced by breast feeding, increased by overcrowding, and linked to the number and age of other siblings, their presence in the same room at night, respiratory infection among them, and parental smoking.[21-23] Domestic air pollution may also affect infant respiratory infection, though the balance of evidence suggests that the effect is small.[24]

Among adults cigarette smoking is the most important known determinant of chronic bronchitis.[25] Mortality from lung cancer in England and Wales does not, however, correlate with infant respiratory mortality.[17] This suggests that the geographical distribution of smoking differs from that of the determinants of respiratory disease in early childhood. By using current death rates from lung cancer as an indicator of cigarette smoking, the statistical dependence of the distribution of chronic bronchitis on infant respiratory infection and smoking can be explored. The results suggest that, in both men and women, smoking is subordinate to infant respiratory infection in determining the geographical distribution of chronic bronchitis within England and Wales.[17]

TABLE 7.1—*Standardised mortality ratios for chronic bronchitis and lung cancer in 10 141 men according to birthweight and weight at one year*

Weight (lb)*	SMR for chronic bronchitis	SMR for lung cancer
Birthweight		
≤5·5	104 (7)	116 (19)
−6·5	86 (16)	64 (30)
−7·5	65 (28)	75 (80)
−8·5	53 (25)	79 (92)
−9·5	72 (17)	57 (33)
>9·5	52 (6)	94 (26)
Weight at one year		
≤18·0	89 (8)	98 (21)
−20·0	89 (23)	89 (56)
−22·0	70 (33)	73 (86)
−24·0	61 (25)	58 (59)
−26·0	44 (9)	92 (46)
>26·0	14 (1)	66 (12)
All	66 (99)	75 (280)

Numbers of deaths in parentheses.
*1 lb = 454 g.

Follow up studies

Direct evidence of a link between lower respiratory tract infection in early childhood and chronic bronchitis has come from two recent follow up studies in the counties of Hertfordshire and Derbyshire, England.[26 27] In both places records of health visitors from the early years of this century have been preserved. Health visitors had visited each child born in the county periodically throughout infancy and early childhood, and noted the occurrence of illnesses. In Hertfordshire, the babies' birthweights and weights at one year of age were also recorded.

In an initial study of 5700 men born in Hertfordshire during 1911–30, death rates from chronic bronchitis fell from those with low to those with high birthweights and weights at one year of age.[26] Table 7.1 shows more recent results for the full cohort of 10 141 men (unpublished data). Standardised mortality ratios fall from 104 in men of birthweight 5·5 lb or less (≤2·5 kg) to 52 in men of birthweight more than 9·5 lb (>4·3 kg). There is a stronger trend with weight at one year of age, standardised mortality ratios falling from 89 in men who weighed 18 lb or less (≤8·2 kg) to 14 in men who weighed more than 26 lb (>11·8 kg). There is no similar trend in death rates for lung cancer. Rates of chronic bronchitis are lower in women, and there are too few deaths to be studied usefully. The relationship between death from chronic bronchitis and weight at one year of age in men (table 7.1) suggests that it may be the disproportionately short baby (see fig 3.9) who fails to grow in infancy who develops chronic

TABLE 7.2—*Mean forced expiratory volume in one second (FEV$_1$) (litres) adjusted for height and age among men aged 59–70 years according to birthweight and smoking habit*

Birthweight (lb)*	Non-smokers	Ex-smokers	Current smokers	All
≤5·5	2·53 (4)	2·34 (16)	2·14 (13)	2·28 (33)
−6·5	2·48 (20)	2·46 (52)	2·29 (31)	2·41 (103)
−7·5	2·65 (37)	2·49 (154)	2·21 (67)	2·44 (258)
−8·5	2·77 (39)	2·53 (134)	2·35 (69)	2·52 (242)
−9·5	2·83 (19)	2·60 (75)	2·30 (38)	2·55 (132)
>9·5	2·79 (8)	2·60 (31)	2·43 (18)	2·57 (57)
All	2·69 (127)	2·52 (462)	2·29 (236)	2·48 (825)†
p value for trend				0·0007

*1 lb = 454 g.
†Standard deviation = 0·59.
Numbers of men in parentheses.

bronchitis. A preliminary study of FEV$_1$ (forced expiratory volume in 1 second) values among 50-year-old men and women in Preston supports this (unpublished data).

The lung function of a sample of 825 men was measured.[26] Their mean FEV$_1$ rose from those with low to those with high birthweight (table 7.2). The effect of birthweight on FEV$_1$, which was strongly statistically significant, was independent of the effect of current height, and almost half as strong. FEV$_1$ was not related to weight at one year, independent of birthweight, which suggests that it is associated with growth *in utero* rather than with growth during infancy. A link to fetal rather than to early postnatal growth might be expected because growth of the airways is largely completed *in utero*.[28] A study of children has also shown that low birthweight is associated with a lower FEV$_1$.[29] These findings suggest that retarded weight gain *in utero* is associated with a constraint on the growth of the airways which is never made up.

As would be expected, men who smoked had a lower FEV$_1$ than those who did not smoke. Table 7.2 shows that the trend of increasing FEV$_1$ with increasing birthweight occurred in men who had never smoked (non-smokers), in ex-smokers, and in current smokers. The trend also occurred at each level of social class. In contrast to FEV$_1$ the forced vital capacity (FVC) was not related to birthweight but was reduced in men with lower weights at one year of age. An interpretation of this is that aspects of lung physiology which determine FVC, as opposed to FEV$_1$, are programmed in infancy rather than during intrauterine life. This interpretation is supported by a study of seven-year-old children whose FVC was not related to birthweight but whose FEV$_1$ was.[30]

In 1923 the health visitors in Hertfordshire began to visit children, after infancy, up to five years of age when they went to school. Tables 7.3 and 7.4 show FEV$_1$ and FVC values for the 639 men born from 1923 onwards, 59 of whom were recorded as having had an attack of bronchitis or

TABLE 7.3—*Mean forced expiratory volume in one second (FEV₁), litres, adjusted for height and age among men aged 59–67 years according to birthweight and the occurrence of bronchitis or pneumonia in infancy*

Birthweight (lb)*	Bronchitis or pneumonia in infancy	
	Absent	Present
≤5·5	2·39 (22)	1·81 (4)
−6·5	2·40 (70)	2·23 (10)
−7·5	2·47 (163)	2·38 (25)
−8·5	2·53 (179)	2·33 (12)
−9·5	2·54 (103)	2·36 (5)
>9·5	2·57 (43)	2·36 (3)
All	2·50 (580)	2·30 (59)

*1 lb = 454 g.
Numbers of men in parentheses.

TABLE 7.4—*Mean forced vital capacity (FVC), litres, adjusted for height and age among men aged 59–67 years according to birthweight and the occurrence of bronchitis or pneumonia in infancy*

Birthweight (lb)*	Bronchitis or pneumonia in infancy	
	Absent	Present
≤5·5	2·91 (22)	2·88 (4)
−6·5	3·02 (70)	2·81 (10)
−7·5	2·94 (163)	2·74 (25)
−8·5	3·03 (179)	2·76 (12)
−9·5	3·01 (103)	2·75 (5)
>9·5	3·11 (43)	2·57 (3)
All	3·00 (580)	2·76 (59)

*1 lb = 454 g.
Numbers of men in parentheses.

pneumonia during infancy. At each birthweight their mean FEV_1 and FVC values were lower than those of men not recorded as having had bronchitis or pneumonia. Sixty three men were recorded as having had an attack of bronchitis or pneumonia between one and five years of age, but their mean FEV_1 and FVC values were similar to those of all the other men. Lower respiratory tract infection before the age of one year was associated with reduced lung function, independent of birthweight, smoking habit, and social class.

Shaheen and colleagues provided further evidence of the long term effects of respiratory infection in early life in a study of 70-year-old men in Derbyshire, England, which also made use of health visitors' records.[27] The FEV_1 of men who had had pneumonia before the age of two years was 0·65 litre less than that of other men, a reduction in FEV_1 of approximately twice that associated with life-long smoking.

The simplest explanation of these observations is that infection of the lower respiratory tract during a critical period in infancy has persisting deleterious effects. Taussig has proposed an alternative explanation, however, namely that occurrence of lower respiratory infection in infancy plays no part in the causation of chronic bronchitis but merely identifies people in whom airway growth is constrained in early life and who are therefore more likely to develop symptoms if infection occurs.[31] According to this explanation, symptomatic lower respiratory tract infection identifies people in whom impaired lung function has already been programmed *in utero*. Prospective studies of children whose lung function has been measured soon after birth may help to resolve this.[32]

GROWTH OF THE LUNG

Whatever the outcome of these studies, lung growth *in utero* seems to have a major effect on chronic bronchitis in adult life. In humans, airway division down to the level of the terminal bronchioles is completed by week 16 of gestation.[28] This is followed by a rapid period of lung growth, so that between 17 and 20 weeks the lung cell population doubles. At 20 weeks the lungs are twice as large relative to the body weight as at term.[33] Alveoli can be detected as early as 30 weeks in the fetus.[34 35] Early studies suggested that around 10% of the adult number of alveoli are present at birth,[36 37] but more recent studies suggest that this is a considerable underestimate.[35 38] Around 50% of the adult alveoli may be present at birth, although there is wide variation. After birth, multiplication slows and is almost complete by two years of age, although during this period there is a rapid increase in alveolar size and complexity.[38] Ninety five per cent of the adult alveolar surface is formed postnatally.[35] In childhood the airway size may be inferred from measures of flow.[39 40] Longitudinal studies suggest that airway growth "tracks" through childhood and that the trajectory of growth is established before the age of one year.[41 42]

Adverse influences may impair airway growth or enhance alveolar growth, depending on their nature and timing, and lead to airflow obstruction, as indicated by a reduction in the ratio of FEV_1/FVC. Undernutrition in mid–late gestation is likely to impair airway growth, leading to a reduced FEV_1. Alveolar growth may, however, be stimulated by hypoxia leading to an increase in FVC. This is known to occur in animals and seems to occur in humans born at altitude.[43]

The frequency of lung hypoplasia at postmortem examination of aborted fetuses or babies who died perinatally suggests that lung growth *in utero* is often impaired.[44] Reduced intrauterine growth is associated with persisting abnormalities of lung function in childhood. Within a group of children who weighed less than 2000 grams at birth, most of whom were pre-term, lower birthweight was associated with a lower FEV_1, adjusted for height, at the age of seven years.[30] In a larger study of children aged 5–11 years, those with lower birthweight had a lower FEV_1, allowing for age and height and independently of the duration of gestation.[29]

The pattern of early lung growth differs in boys and girls: in boys airway growth tends to lag behind parenchymal growth.[39] Boys have a larger lung volume than girls of a similar age and stature, but longer narrower airways in relation to that volume.[38 45] In the Hertfordshire study, the associations between birthweight and FEV_1 were weaker in women (unpublished data) and this could be explained by sex differences in early lung growth. In a similar way, the associations between lower respiratory tract infection in early childhood and FEV_1 were weaker in women in Hertfordshire and Derbyshire.[27] This is consistent with the results of a study of children in whom pneumonia in early childhood was related to impaired lung function in boys but not in girls.[46] Boys are known to have more severe lower respiratory tract infection than girls in infancy, and they are more likely to be hospitalised with bronchiolitis.[47 48] This has been attributed partly to the smaller airway size.[40]

Conclusions

In the past, discussion of the natural history of chronic bronchitis tended to focus on the rate of decline of adult lung function.[49] The findings described here, however, suggest the disease is associated with impaired lung growth in early life. Influences which determine the rate of functional decline, of which smoking is the most important, add to the effects of impaired early growth.

Green has suggested that the susceptibility to smoking damage may be linked to the pattern of lung growth and structure.[50] A moderate smoker who failed to attain maximal lung function potential as a young adult may develop chronic bronchitis at the same age as a heavy smoker who achieved maximal lung growth.[4] The findings in Hertfordshire suggest that the effects of poor growth and smoking on lung function are additive and not synergistic, although measures of early body weight may be poor indicators of lung growth. To test this more rigorously it will be necessary to relate early growth to the longitudinal rate of decline in FEV_1 in smokers and non-smokers.

Thinking on the pathogenesis of emphysema has been dominated by a destructive model involving protease–antiprotease balance.[51] Developmental models, such as those produced in animals, may be more relevant.[52]

Summary

The hypothesis that lower respiratory tract infection during infancy causes chronic bronchitis in adult life is supported by the similar geographical distribution of the two disorders. Follow up studies have shown that low growth rates *in utero* and during infancy, and early respiratory infection, predict abnormal lung function and disease in adult life. The effects of cigarette smoking in adult life add to those occurring in early life. Airway growth *in utero* may have an important effect on chronic bronchitis. Infection of the lower respiratory tract in infancy may also have persistent deleterious effects or may simply identify children in whom airway growth has been constrained *in utero*.

1 Orie NGM, Sluiter HJ, eds. *Bronchitis—an international symposium*. Groningen, the Netherlands: Assen Royal Vengorium, 1961.
2 Holland WW, Halil T, Bennett AE, Elliott A. Factors influencing the onset of chronic respiratory disease. *BMJ* 1969;**ii**:205–8.
3 Reid DD. The beginnings of bronchitis. *Proceedings of the Royal Society of Medicine* 1969;**62**:311–16.
4 Samet JM, Tager IB, Speizer FE. The relationship between respiratory illness in childhood and chronic airflow obstruction in adulthood. *Am Rev Respir Dis* 1983;**127**:508–23.
5 Phelan PD. Does adult chronic obstructive lung disease really begin in childhood? *Br J Dis Chest* 1984;**78**:1–9.
6 Strachan DP. Do chesty children become chesty adults? *Arch Dis Child* 1990;**65**:161–2.
7 Reid DD, Fletcher CM. International studies in chronic respiratory disease. *Br Med Bull* 1971;**27**:59–64.
8 Osmond C, Barker DJP, Slattery JM. Risk of death from cardiovascular disease and chronic bronchitis determined by place of birth in England and Wales. *J Epidemiol Community Health* 1990;**44**:139–41.
9 Kattan M, Keens TG, Lapierre JG, Levison H, Bryan AC, Reilly BJ. Pulmonary function abnormalities in symptom-free children after bronchiolitis. *Pediatrics* 1977;**59**:683–8.
10 Gurwitz D, Mindorff C, Levison H. Increased incidence of bronchial reactivity in children with a history of bronchiolitis. *Pediatrics* 1981;**98**:551–5.
11 Pullan CR, Hey EN. Wheezing, asthma and pulmonary dysfunction 10 years after infection with respiratory syncytial virus in infancy. *BMJ* 1982;**284**:1665–9.
12 Mok JYQ, Simpson H. Outcome for acute bronchitis, bronchiolitis, and pneumonia in infancy. *Arch Dis Child* 1984;**59**:306–9.
13 Kiernan KE, Colley JRT, Douglas JWB, Reid DD. Chronic cough in young adults in relation to smoking habits, childhood environment and chest illness. *Respiration* 1976;**33**:236–44.
14 Britten N, Davies JMC, Colley JRT. Early respiratory experience and subsequent cough and peak expiratory flow rate in 36 year old men and women. *BMJ* 1987;**294**:1317–20.
15 Mann SL, Wadsworth MEJ, Colley JRT. Accumulation of factors influencing respiratory illness in members of a national birth cohort and their offspring. *J Epidemiol Community Health* 1992;**46**:286–92.
16 Gardner MJ, Winter PD, Barker DJP. *Atlas of mortality from selected diseases in England and Wales*. 1968–78. Chichester: Wiley, 1984.

17 Barker DJP, Osmond C. Childhood respiratory infection and adult chronic bronchitis in England and Wales. *BMJ* 1986;**293**:1271–5.

18 Registrar General. Statistical review of England and Wales. Part I: tables, medical. London: HMSO, 1911 *et seq.*

19 Boyd JT. Climate, air pollution and mortality. *Br J Prev Soc Med* 1960;**14**:123–35.

20 Colley JRT. Respiratory disease in childhood. *Br Med Bull* 1971;**27**:9–14.

21 Downham MAPS, Scott R, Sims DG, Webb JKG, Gardner PS. Breast feeding protects against respiratory syncytial virus infections. *BMJ* 1976;**ii**:274–6.

22 Leeder SR, Corkhill R, Irwig LM, Holland WW, Colley JRT. Influence of family factors on the incidence of lower respiratory illness during the first year of life. *Br J Prev Soc Med* 1976;**30**:203–12.

23 Pullan CR, Toms GL, Martin AG, Gardner PS, Webb JKG, Appleton DR. Breast feeding and respiratory syncytial virus infection. *BMJ* 1980;**281**:1034–8.

24 Ogston SA, Florey C du V, Walker CHM. The Tayside infant morbidity and mortality study: effect on health of using gas for cooking. *BMJ* 1985;**290**:957–60.

25 Lambert PM, Reid DD. Smoking, air pollution, and bronchitis in Britain. *Lancet* 1970; **i**:853–7.

26 Barker DJP, Godfrey KM, Fall C, Osmond C, Winter PD, Shaheen SO. Relation of birthweight and childhood respiratory infection to adult lung function and death from chronic obstructive airways disease. *BMJ* 1991;**303**:671–5.

27 Shaheen SO, Barker DJP, Shiell AW, Crocker FJ, Wield GA, Holgate ST. The relationship between pneumonia in early childhood and impaired lung function in late adult life. *Am J Respir Crit Care Med* 1994;**149**:616–19.

28 Bucher U, Reid L. Development of the intrasegmental bronchial tree; the pattern of branching and development of cartilage at various stages of intrauterine life. *Thorax* 1961;**16**:207–18.

29 Rona RJ, Gulliford MC, Chinn S. Effects of prematurity and intrauterine growth on respiratory health and lung function in childhood. *BMJ* 1993;**306**:817–20.

30 Chan KN, Noble-Jamieson CM, Elliman A, Bryan EM, Silverman M. Lung function in children of low birth weight. *Arch Dis Child* 1989;**64**:1284–93.

31 Taussig LM. The conundrum of wheezing and airway hyperreactivity in infancy. *Pediatr Pulmonol* 1992;**13**:1–3.

32 Martinez FD, Morgan WJ, Wright AL, Holberg C, Taussig LM. Initial airway function is a risk factor for recurrent wheezing respiratory illnesses during the first three years of life. *Am Rev Respir Dis* 1991;**143**:312–16.

33 Wigglesworth JS, Desai R. Use of DNA estimation for growth assessment in normal and hypoplastic fetal lungs. *Arch Dis Child* 1981;**56**:601–5.

34 Langston C, Kida K, Reed M, Thurlbeck WM. Human lung growth in late gestation and in the neonate. *Am Rev Respir Dis* 1984;**129**:607–13.

35 Hislop AA, Wigglesworth JS, Desai R. Alveolar development in the human fetus and infant. *Early Human Development* 1986;**13**:1–11.

36 Dunnill MS. Postnatal growth of the lung. *Thorax* 1962;**17**:329–33.

37 Davies G, Reid L. Growth of the alveoli and pulmonary arteries in childhood. *Thorax* 1970;**25**:669–81.

38 Thurlbeck WM. Postnatal human lung growth. *Thorax* 1982;**37**:564–71.

39 Pagtakhan RD, Bjelland JC, Landau LI, *et al.* Sex differences in growth patterns of the airways and lung parenchyma in children. *J Appl Physiol* 1984;**56**:1204–10.

40 Tepper RS, Morgan WJ, Cota K, *et al.* Physiologic growth and development of the lung during the first year of life. *Am Rev Respir Dis* 1986;**134**:513–19.

41 Dockery DW, Berkey CS, Ware JH, Speizer FE, Ferris BG Jr. Distribution of forced vital capacity and forced expiratory volume in one second in children 6 to 11 years of age. *Am Rev Respir Dis* 1983;**128**:405–12.

42 Chan KN, Wong YC, Silverman M. Relationship between infant lung mechanics and childhood lung function in children of very low birthweight. *Pediatr Pulmonol* 1990;**8**:74–81.

43 Brody JS, Vaccaro C. Postnatal formation of alveoli: interstitial events and physiologic consequences. *Fed Proc* 1979;**38**:215–23.

44 Wigglesworth JS, Desai R. Is fetal respiratory function a major determinant of perinatal survival? *Lancet* 1982;**i**:264–7.

45 Hibbert ME, Couriel JM, Landau LI. Changes in lung, airway and chest wall function in boys and girls between 8 and 12 years. *J Appl Physiol* 1984;**57**:304–8.

46 Gold DR, Tager IB, Weiss ST, Tosteson TD, Speizer FE. Acute lower respiratory illness in childhood as a predictor of lung function and chronic respiratory symptoms. *Am Rev Respir Dis* 1989;**140**:877–84.

47 Glezen WP, Denny FW. Epidemiology of acute lower respiratory disease in children. *N Engl J Med* 1973;**288**:498–505.

48 Breese Hall C. Respiratory syncytial virus. In: Feigin RD, Cherry JD, eds, *Textbook of pediatric infectious diseases*. Philadelphia: WB Saunders, 1981:1247–66.

49 Burrows B. Natural history of chronic airflow obstruction. In: Hensley MJ, Saunders NA, eds, *Clinical epidemiology of chronic obstructive pulmonary disease. Lung biology in health and disease*, vol 43. New York: Marcel Dekker, 1989: 99–107.

50 Green M, Mead J, Turner JM. Variability of maximum expiratory flow-volume curves. *J Appl Physiol* 1974,**37**:67–74.

51 Janoff A. State of the art. Elastases and emphysema: current assessment of the protease-antiprotease hypothesis. *Am Rev Respir Dis* 1985;**132**:417–33.

52 O'Dell BL, Kilburn KH, McKenzie WN, Thurston RJ. The lung of the copper-deficient rat. *Am J Pathol* 1978;**91**:413–32.

8: Infection after birth and disease in later life

Persistent effects of lower respiratory tract infection during infancy are immediately apparent. Bronchiolitis, bronchitis, and pneumonia are often followed by cough, wheeze, and impaired lung function which persist through childhood. Effects of other infections in early childhood, however, are not immediately apparent. There may be a prolonged latent period before disorders develop in middle or late life. "Shingles" (herpes zoster), a disease of later life caused by infection with the chickenpox virus during childhood, is a familiar example.

A number of diseases have recently been identified as possible delayed consequences of early infection. This chapter takes as examples two diseases, acute appendicitis and Paget's disease of bone.

Acute appendicitis

Acute appendicitis occurs at all ages but is most common during childhood and adolescence.

TIME TRENDS

A striking feature of the epidemiology of the disease is its time trends. Fig 8.1 shows average annual mortality rates for appendicitis in England and Wales since 1901, when the disease was first recognised as an entity by the Registrar General.[1] In medical journals at the beginning of the century, there was considerable correspondence about the disease and general agreement that the increase in Britain began around 1890–95. The disease was recognised and described long before that but was seemingly rare.[2] Anecdotal evidence and analysis of hospital records suggest that the rise began abruptly.[3-5] There is evidence of a similarly abrupt rise in Germany, in the French army, and in Russia.[6-8]

It is probable that during the first two decades of the century incidence rates rose more steeply than death rates because case fatality fell sharply. The rise may, however, have been exaggerated by wider recognition of the disease. Probably the constant mortality during the 1920s reflected rising incidence and falling case fatality.[1 9 10] There are no incidence data for the

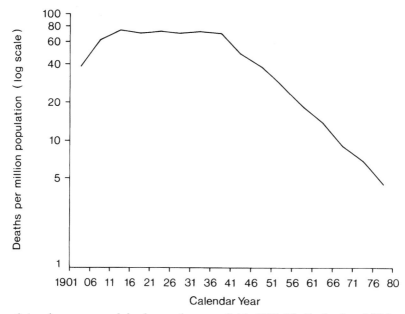

FIG 8.1—*Average annual death rates for appendicitis 1901–80, England and Wales.*

general population but National Health Insurance statistics for Scotland during 1931–35 indicate a remarkably high annual incidence of around 55 per 10 000, equivalent to a cumulative rate of 5% of the population over 10 years.[9]

During the 1930s death rates began to fall. Examination of age specific trends by single year, rather than the five year averages shown in fig 8.1, shows that in all age groups except the very elderly death rates were already declining when the Second World War began (fig 8.2). From 1940 onwards the rate of fall did not change greatly, and the decline continued almost without interruption through the post-war years. In the USA there was also a decline in mortality during the 1930s.[9] Hospital discharge rates in Britain, general practitioner consultation rates, and a local survey confirm that the post-war decline in mortality reflected a large and continuing decline in incidence.[11–14] A post-war decline in incidence has also been recorded in other European countries and in the USA.[15–19]

The upsurge of the disease from around 1895 may have been exaggerated by more widespread recognition. Its decline, as reflected in mortality, may have been accelerated by changing diagnostic practices in patients with abdominal pain, changing criteria for appendicectomy, and falling case fatality. Nevertheless the overall pattern is clear: a steep rise which began abruptly around 1895 and a steep fall from the 1930s onwards.

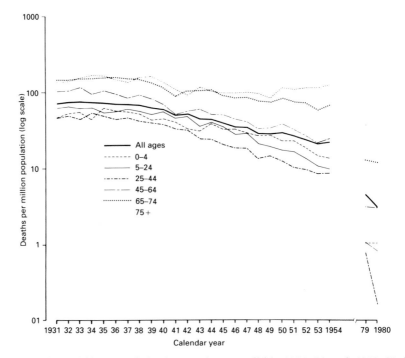

FIG 8.2—*Age specific annual death rates for appendicitis 1931–54 and 1979–80 in England and Wales.*

SOCIAL CLASS

When appendicitis first appeared in Britain it was noted to be more common among children of the rich.[5] These observations were supported by the higher mortality in social classes I and II.[9] Among recruits into the army in the Second World War there were astonishing differences in appendicectomy rates according to social origins. These must have reflected differences in access to medical care as well as incidence of the disease. Since the Second World War the social class gradient in appendicectomy has disappeared.[19]

GEOGRAPHY

In 1910, Owen Williams[20] reviewed the world distribution of the disease. His findings, later extended by Murray[3] and Rendle Short,[4] showed that although it occurred throughout the world it was predominantly a disease of industrialised countries. In non-industrialised countries it was seen only among European residents. More recently, although it remains rare in some areas such as rural sub-Saharan Africa, acute appendicitis is now commonly

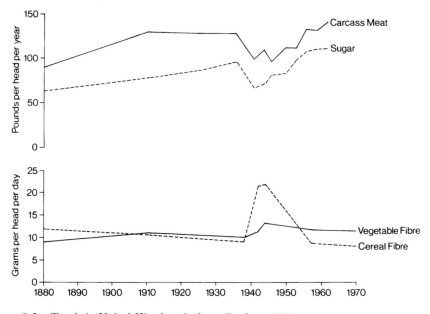

FIG 8.3—*Trends in United Kingdom food supplies from 1880.*

seen in some parts of non-industrialised countries, and findings among Inuit communities support the idea that it has arisen in these areas in association with changes in the way of life.[21]

DIET

In 1920 Rendle Short[4] reviewed the rise of appendicitis in Britain during the previous 20 years and the international differences in its frequency. He concluded that the disease had arisen as a result of "the relatively less quantity of cellulose eaten on account of the wider use of imported foods". From this conclusion arose the "dietary fibre hypothesis" which Burkitt and Trowell later extended to include a range of diseases commonly seen in Western societies.[22-24] Fig 8.3, showing trends in consumption of cereal and vegetable fibre, meat, and sugar since 1880, is based on national estimates of food supplies and consumption in Britain.[25 26] Consumption of meat, sugar, and vegetable fibre increased whereas cereal fibre consumption decreased. These trends were interrupted by the Second World War when introduction of food rationing in 1942 led to a sharp fall in intakes of meat and sugar and a rise in fibre intake, especially cereal fibre which was present in large amounts in the wheat flour used from 1942 to 1953.

Clearly the decline in appendicitis from 1930 onwards does not correlate with changes in fibre, meat, or sugar. Moreover, fig 8.2 gives little support to the conclusion that the decline was initiated by the major changes in the British diet during the Second World War.[27 28] Nor does fig 8.2 suggest that a decline which had already begun was accelerated during wartime.

If the large rise in incidence, from rarity to around 50 cases per 10 000 population per year, was the effect of changing levels of consumption of a particular food, the new levels must be associated with a high risk, both absolute and relative to that in the population before the change. Given the variations among individual diets which still exist within the population, a food associated at certain levels of consumption with a high risk of disease should be readily identified by comparison of the diets of cases of appendicitis with those of controls. This has not proved to be so; the results of case control studies have been inconclusive.[29–31]

If changes in consumption of a food caused the upsurge of appendicitis, the 1880 consumption levels must be regarded as thresholds above which (for fibre) or below which (for meat or sugar) the disease is rarely induced. Such an interpretation, however, is not consistent with the trends during and after the Second World War. At that time both cereal and vegetable fibre consumption were appreciably above the 1880 levels, and meat and sugar consumption fell to levels close to those in 1880. Given a latent period of no more than a few years, at least in children, these dietary changes would be predicted to cause a sharp drop in appendicitis in the 1940s, followed by a rise in incidence in the 1950s when food rationing ceased. There is no evidence that this occurred.

It may be concluded that dietary changes during the past century do not offer a sufficient explanation for either the rise or the decline of appendicitis in Britain. In particular, a close dependence on dietary fibre intake, postulated 60 years ago, and the origin of the hypothesis linking fibre to a range of "Western diseases", does not withstand critical examination of trends. Nevertheless, although dietary changes do not explain the changing incidence of the disease, comparisons of food consumption and rates of acute appendicitis in different areas of Britain and Ireland do suggest that green vegetables may protect against the disease, possibly by changing the bacterial flora of the appendix.[32]

INFECTION

The structure of the appendix is similar to that of other parts of the gut. It has a muscular coat, and a thick submucosal layer distended with lymphatic tissue which tends to encroach on the lumen and make it somewhat small. This lymphatic tissue resembles the tonsil, and may protect the ecosystem of the large intestine from bacteria and viruses. Residue from the small intestine may be diverted into the appendix and sampled by the lymphoid tissue, which may then respond by secreting specific antibodies.[33]

In 1932 Aschoff[8] showed that the ultimate event in appendicitis was invasion of the distal appendicular wall by organisms habitually present among the enteric flora. This remains the general view,[34] and debate centres on the preceding pathological changes. In 1946 Bohrod[35] argued that the initiating event in appendicitis was lymphoid hyperplasia in the appendicular wall and consequent obstruction of the proximal lumen. He pointed out that this would explain the remarkably constant age distribution of the disease in different times and places, because the bulk of lymphoid tissue in the appendicular wall in relation to luminal size is maximal during childhood and adolescence and declines thereafter. The theory also explains the absence of faecoliths, an alternative possible cause of luminal obstruction, in most removed appendices.[23]

The appendicitis epidemic in Britain started at the time when infections had begun to decline steeply, in consequence of improved living standards and sanitation.[36] It may be postulated that decreased incidence of infection among children, especially in wealthier families, changed their patterns of immunity so that they responded to certain enteric or respiratory infections with lymphoid hyperplasia—which included the lymphoid tissue in the wall of the appendix. This changed pathogenic response to infections with a declining frequency in early childhood would be analogous to the age dependent consequences of infection with the poliomyelitis virus. The incidence of poliomyelitis rises as hygiene improves because the central nervous system becomes increasingly vulnerable to it as the age when it is first encountered rises. The association between the Epstein–Barr virus and glandular fever is similarly age dependent.

The so called "hygiene hypothesis" is able to explain the international distribution of appendicitis. Countries where it is common are characterised by lower incidences of infectious disease. The rising incidence of appendicitis among the more affluent, urbanised communities within non-industrialised countries is explained by the improvement in the hygienic conditions of these communities.

Findings in a national sample of 5362 people born in Britain in 1946, at around the peak of the appendicitis epidemic, support the hypothesis.[19] Those born in households with hot water systems and bathrooms had higher rates of appendicitis. The relative risk was 1·0 for those in households with a bathroom compared with 0·7 in those in households without. Those born in less crowded households, that is, with fewer people per room, also had higher rates of appendicitis, but the differences were not statistically significant. This suggested that provision of domestic hot water systems and bathrooms may have been the early change in the transition to "Western" hygiene that caused appendicitis rates to rise in Britain.

Evidence to support this comes from studies in Hong Kong and in the island of Anglesey, Wales. The remarkable improvements in housing, water supplies, and sanitation in Hong Kong since the Second World War have been associated with a steep rise in appendicitis. In a case control comparison Donnan[37] showed that patients with appendicitis had had more household amenities and less crowding in early childhood. Records of operating rooms maintained by the hospitals serving Anglesey over the last 50 years show a sharp rise in rates of appendicitis after the introduction of a piped water supply after the Second World War, and the increase in domestic hot water systems and fixed baths which followed.[38] Provision of piped water to the people of Anglesey was delayed because water sources were scarce and the population was scattered. The appendicitis epidemic in Anglesey occurred while appendicitis rates were falling elsewhere in Britain. Although rates in Anglesey have begun to fall sharply in the last 15 years they remain high, at levels found, in the British Isles, in only the northern and western regions of Ireland and in the Isle of Man.[39 40]

The Anglesey studies suggest that appendicitis rates depend more on the provision of hot water systems and fixed baths than on other household amenities such as piped water and water closets.[38] It is interesting that, in Northern Ireland in 1956, before widespread poliomyelitis immunisation, the antibody status of children was not related to whether the house had a piped water supply. There was, however, a strong association between seropositivity and absence of a hot water system, independent of social class.[41] In Anglesey, before the Second World War, domestic crowding was unusually severe, being remarked on in national surveys.[42] A study of 1900 men and women born on the island during 1932–62 suggested that the fall in crowding levels between 1930 and 1950, which occurred as a result of the falling birth rate and improved housing, may have contributed to the rise in appendicitis rates, independent of the effects of domestic hot water systems.[43]

The hygiene hypothesis—an explanation for the rise and fall of appendicitis

The "hygiene hypothesis" proposes two phases in the incidence of appendicitis.[1] When hygiene begins to improve in a community levels of infection in infants fall. This increases their susceptibility to enteric infection at later ages, perhaps through more vigorous lymphoid hyperplasia in the appendicular wall with consequent luminal obstruction. As hygiene continues to improve, however, exposure to enteric infections which trigger acute appendicitis is reduced further, and appendicitis declines. The occurrence of appendicitis has been recorded in two national samples of British children who were born in 1958 and 1970, when appendicitis rates were declining. In each of the cohorts children were more at risk of appendicectomy if they lived in households that lacked amenities and where they were therefore more exposed to enteric infections. A geographical study of appendicitis in Ireland in 1980 similarly showed that rates were higher where fewer households had fixed baths and hot water systems.[32] In a study in Anglesey Coggon showed that the greatest risk of appendicitis was among people who were born in houses with amenities and then moved to houses without them.[43] The hygiene hypothesis illustrates how the incidence of a disease may rise and fall in response to one continuing environmental change. This is important because when "Western diseases" such as appendicitis appear in response to industrialisation and the accompanying changes in way of life it is often argued that their prevention necessarily depends upon a return to practices of the past. This theme is developed in chapter 11.

Paget's disease of bone

James Paget's[44] original description of this disease in 1876 was of an elderly gentleman with progressive skeletal deformities. Subsequent clinical, postmortem examination and radiological case series showed that the disease is more prevalent among men than women.[45 46] It is most common in elderly people although many young patients have been described, symptoms sometimes beginning in the early twenties.

TIME TRENDS

In Britain death rates from Paget's disease have declined markedly during the last 40 years. Fig 8.4 shows that if rates are analysed so that they show the mortality experience of successive generations, or cohorts, those born from around 1880 onwards had progressively lower death rates at any particular age. Generation analysis of mortality from Paget's disease in Scotland and among white people in the USA reveals a similar pattern, although the US rates are lower throughout.[47] If mortality from Paget's disease is accepted as an indicator of its incidence, then an inference is that successive generations have been exposed less and less to some aetiological influence. The existence of strong generation effects is consistent with the disease originating through exposure to an environmental influence in early life. Coronary heart disease and stroke show such effects, which are discussed further in chapter 11.

GEOGRAPHY

Although isolated case reports have come from many parts of the world, clinical observations suggest that the disease is common only in Europe, North America, Australia, and New Zealand.[48] Perhaps the most remarkable feature of the disease's geography is the variation in rates within Europe. In a survey in western Europe the prevalence of the disease was mapped from replies to a postal questionnaire completed by radiologists in 13 countries.[49] The questionnaire enquired about the frequency with which Paget's disease was seen, as either the principal abnormality or, more often, an incidental one. The questionnaire was validated by replies from radiologists in Britain, where the radiological prevalence had already been measured (as will be described), and in Norway, where there was previous

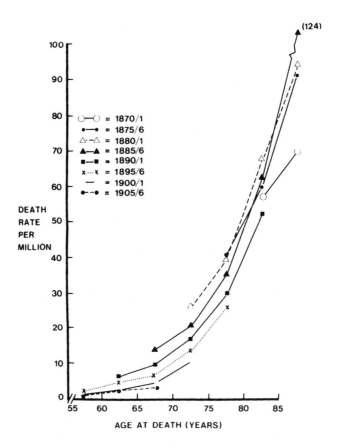

FIG 8.4—*Cohort mortality from Paget's disease in England and Wales in five year periods, 1951–75.*

evidence of a low prevalence.[50] The responses showed a clear pattern. The disease was most common in Britain, less common in France, and beyond France the frequency declined to the south, east, and north-east. The disease was rare in Scandinavia.

More precise information, which corroborated that obtained from the postal questionnaire, came from a series of radiological surveys measuring the prevalence of clinical and subclinical disease.[49 51] The results of surveys carried out in 15 European towns are shown in fig 8.5. The prevalence shown for Britain is the mean for 31 towns surveyed.[47 51] Outside Britain the highest prevalences were found in three French towns: Bordeaux (2·7%), Rennes (2·4%), and Nancy (2·0%). These prevalences were lower than the overall prevalence of 4·6% in Britain, but were comparable with the lowest values recorded in individual towns there. In the remaining

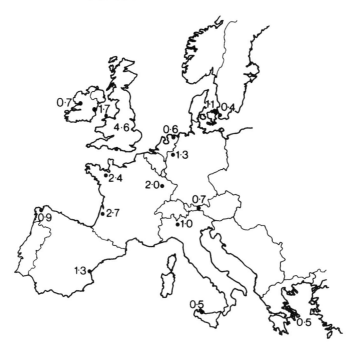

FIG 8.5—*Prevalence (%) of Paget's disease among men and women aged 55 years and over in 15 European towns and in Britain.*

European towns, the prevalences ranged from 1·7% in Dublin, and 1·3% in Valencia (Spain) and Essen (Germany), to 0·5% in Palermo (Sicily) and Athens, and 0·4% in Malmo (Sweden). The low prevalence in Dublin (1·7%), situated so close to Britain, is remarkable, as is the rarity of the disease in western Ireland (0·7% in Galway).

The survey of 31 towns in Britain revealed a localised area of high prevalence. The six towns with the highest prevalences (ranging from 6·3% to 8·3% compared with the national average of 5·0%) were all situated within a small area of the county of Lancashire.[51] Outside this area the rates fell away sharply, with the bordering towns having prevalences of around the average for all towns. (The national average of 5·0% in this study, compared with 4·6% shown in fig 8.5, reflects exclusion of radiographs taken specifically to investigate skeletal disease from the European Study.[49]) More recently a focus of high prevalence has been found in La Cabrera, in Spain.[52]

MIGRANTS

Within the USA comparison of a northern city, New York, with Atlanta, in the south, showed a marked difference, with prevalences among white

TABLE 8.1—*Prevalence of Paget's disease by ethnic group in two American cities*

City	Ethnic group	No.of radiographs	Age standardised prevalence (%) Men	Women	Both sexes
New York	Black	950	3·3 (12)	2·0 (12)	2·6 (24)
New York	White	1082	5·2 (30)	2·5 (13)	3·9 (43)
Atlanta	Black	1111	1·9 (11)	0·6 (3)	1·2 (14)
Atlanta	White	1563	0·9 (7)	0·8 (6)	0·9 (13)

Figures in parentheses are numbers of cases.

people being 3·9% in New York and only 1·9% in Atlanta[53 54] (table 8.1). Markedly lower rates in the southern city were also seen among black people. It is interesting that the prevalences in black Americans were similar to those among white people, because the disease has rarely been reported in Africa, outside of South Africa, where prevalences in white and black people are also similar. [55 56]

Findings in Australia (table 8.2) parallel those in the USA. The prevalence among British born immigrants (4.0%) was intermediate between the British rate (5·0%) and the rate among native born Australians (3·2%).[57] These two sets of observations among communities that have migrated point strongly to the influence of environment in the aetiology of the disease.

INFECTION

There have been many reports of Paget's disease affecting more than one member of a family, including its occurrence in successive generations.[58] Pedigree studies of the distribution of the disease in selected families once led to the conclusion that it is an autosomal dominant disorder.[59] The epidemiological findings do not, however, support the idea that there is such a clearly defined genetic influence in aetiology. Many hypotheses about environmental causes of Paget's disease, for example, bacterial infection, a toxin, or fluorine poisoning, have arisen and been discarded. Current interest centres on the discovery that the nuclei of osteoclast cells in pagetoid bone contain inclusion bodies whose appearance resembles paramyxovirus nucleocapsides.[60 61] This raises the possibility that the disease

TABLE 8.2—*Prevalence of Paget's disease in Australia and the United Kingdom by place of birth and place of residence*

Place of birth	Place of residence	Age standardised prevalence (%) Men	Women	Both sexes
UK	UK	6·2	3·9	5·0
UK	Australia	5·7	2·3	4·0
Australia	Australia	3·5	2·8	3·2

is the result of infection with a "slow virus", which initiates malfunctioning of osteoclast cells—currently thought to be the primary pathological disorder in the disease. Interest is centred on two particular paramyxoviruses: measles virus and respiratory syncytial virus.

If viral infection is a cause of Paget's disease, the virus must be capable of considerable penetration within populations, for the disease affects up to 8% of people aged 55 and over in British towns. By contrast, its penetration, in so far as this is indicated by the prevalence of the disease, is poor in adjacent populations, notably Ireland and Scandinavia, and in densely populated northern European areas such as Essen in Germany. There is no parallel with any other human viral illness and it seems necessary to postulate the existence of one or more as yet unknown co-factors. Vitamin D deficiency in childhood has been proposed but the evidence is no more than suggestive.[62] Different patterns of age at infection in different countries together with differing long term consequences of infection at different ages is another possibility.

Epidemiological studies have suggested viruses other than measles or respiratory syncytial virus as causes of Paget's disease. A survey in Manchester, England, showed that ownership of dogs in the past was more common among patients with Paget's disease than among controls.[63] This led to the suggestion that a canine virus, possibly canine distemper virus, might be the primary infective agent in the disease. Studies in Spain, Italy, and England failed to confirm this finding.[52 64] Moreover the European distribution of Paget's disease (see fig 8.5) does not parallel the distribution of dogs. Sweden, for example, has 9·6 dogs per 100 people, which is similar to the figure of 10·4 for Britain.

Other diseases

The continuing story of Paget's disease illustrates how the search for the causes of chronic diseases is being refocused on infection in early childhood. Other examples are motor neuron disease and multiple sclerosis. Martyn has proposed that motor neuron disease, which causes progressive muscular weakness in middle to late life, may be an uncommon sequel to poliovirus infection.[65 66] Epidemiological studies support this hypothesis.[67 68] The possibility that multiple sclerosis may be linked to early infection is a recurring theme of the literature because viruses are known to destroy the myelin sheath of nerves, and loss of myelin is the lesion that underlies the disease.[69] There is increasing evidence that patients with multiple sclerosis have had an unusual early experience of infectious disease.[70-73] A number of studies suggest that people with the disease have the common communicable diseases of childhood at a later age than others, and recent findings which link the disease to delayed exposure to the Epstein–Barr virus encourage further exploration of this hypothesis.[74-76]

Summary

Infections in early childhood are suspected to determine a number of diseases in later life, following a prolonged latent period. For example, acute appendicitis may be determined by exposure to infections of the gut after birth, and Paget's disease of bone has been linked to childhood measles. The effects of early infections may depend on the age at which they are first encountered, the likelihood of long term effects being greater at older ages. Age dependent consequences of infection provide a model that could explain why some "Western diseases" such as appendicitis increase in response to industrialisation and then decline. The progressive decline in incidence of other diseases, such as Paget's disease, affects successive generations so that each generation has lower rates at every age. Such "cohort" trends are shown by diseases that are initiated in early life.

1 Barker DJP. Acute appendicitis and dietary fibre: an alternative hypothesis. *BMJ* 1985; **290**:1125–7.
2 Fitz RH. Perforating inflammation of the vermiform appendix: with special reference to its early diagnosis and treatment. *Am J Med Sci* 1886;**92**:321–45.
3 Murray RW. The geographical distribution of appendicitis. *Lancet* 1914;**ii**:227–30.
4 Rendle Short A. The causation of appendicitis. *Br J Surg* 1920;**8**:171–88.
5 Spencer AM. Aetiology of acute appendicitis. *BMJ* 1938;**i**:227–30.
6 Special correspondence. *BMJ* 1903;**i**:1373.
7 Gazeta dos Hospitaes do Porto. Quoted in *BMJ* 1908;**ii**:191.
8 Aschoff L. (Translated by Pether GC.) *Appendicitis, its aetiology and pathology.* London: Constable, 1932.
9 Young M, Russell WT. *Appendicitis, a statistical study. Medical Research Council Special Report Series No 233.* London: HMSO, 1939.
10 Boyce FF. Acute appendicitis and its complications. New York: Oxford University Press, 1949.
11 *Report on the hospital in-patient enquiry.* London: HMSO, 1957 and following years.
12 *Mortality statistics from general practice, studies on medical and population subjects,* Nos 14 and 26. London: HMSO, 1958 and 1975.
13 Donnan SPB, Lambert PM. Appendicitis: incidence and mortality. *Population Trends* 1976;**5**:26–8.
14 Raguveer-Saran MK, Keddie NC. The falling incidence of appendicitis. *Br J Surg* 1980;**67**:681.
15 Lunn-Rockliffe WEC. Army recruits and appendicitis. *BMJ* 1942;**i**:623.
16 Castleton KB, Puestow CB, Sauer D. Is appendicitis decreasing in frequency? *Arch Surg* 1959;**78**:794–801.
17 Palumbo LT. Appendicitis—is it on the wane? *Am J Surg* 1959;**98**:702–3.
18 Arnbjornsson E, Asp NG, Westin SI. Decreasing incidence of acute appendicitis with special reference to the consumption of dietary fiber. *Acta Chir Scand* 1982;**148**: 461–4.
19 Barker DJP, Osmond C, Golding J, Wadsworth MEJ. Acute appendicitis and bathrooms in three samples of British children. *BMJ* 1988;**296**:956–8.

20 Williams OT. The distribution of appendicitis, with some observations on its relation to diet. *BMJ* 1910;**ii**:2016–21.

21 Schaefer O. Aetiology of appendicitis. *BMJ* 1979;**i**:1215.

22 Burkitt DP. The aetiology of appendicitis. *Br J Surg* 1971;**58**:695–9.

23 Trowell HC, Burkitt DP. *Western diseases: their emergence and prevention.* London: Edward Arnold, 1981.

24 Burkitt DP. In: GG Birch, KJ Parker, eds, *Dietary fibre.* London: Applied Science, 1983.

25 Greaves JP, Hollingsworth DF. Trends in food consumption in the United Kingdom. *World Rev Nutr Diet* 1966;**6**:34–89.

26 Southgate DAT, Bingham S, Robertson J. Dietary fibre in the British diet. *Nature* 1978; **274**:51–2.

27 Rendle Short A. *The causation of appendicitis.* Bristol: John Wright, 1946.

28 Donnan SPB. Aetiology of appendicitis. *BMJ* 1979;**i**:1215.

29 Cove-Smith JR, Langman MJS. Appendicitis and dietary fibre. *Gut* 1975;**16**:409.

30 Arnbjornsson E. Acute appendicitis and dietary fiber. *Arch Surg* 1983;**118**:868–70.

31 Nelson M, Morris J, Barker DJP, Simmonds S. A case-control study of acute appendicitis and diet in children. *J Epidemiol Community Health* 1986;**40**:316–18.

32 Barker DJP, Morris J. Acute appendicitis, bathrooms, and diet in Britain and Ireland. *BMJ* 1988;**296**:953–5.

33 Read NW. Pathophysiological mechanisms in the appendix. In: *The aetiology of acute appendicitis.* (Scientific Report No 7.) Southampton: MRC Environmental Epidemiology Unit, 1986:23–6.

34 Pieper R, Kager L, Weintraub A, Lindberg AA, Nord CE. The role of bacteroides fragilis in the pathogenesis of acute appendicitis. *Acta Chir Scand* 1982;**148**:39–44.

35 Bohrod MG. The pathogenesis of acute appendicitis. *Am J Clin Pathol* 1946;**16**:752–60.

36 McKeown T, Lowe CR. *An introduction to social medicine.* Oxford: Blackwell, 1977.

37 Donnan SPB. Appendicitis in Hong Kong. In: *The aetiology of acute appendicitis.* (Scientific Report No 7.) Southampton: MRC Environmental Epidemiology Unit, 1986:16–19.

38 Barker DJP, Morris JA, Simmonds SJ, Oliver RHP. Appendicitis epidemic following introduction of piped water to Anglesey. *J Epidemiol Community Health* 1988;**2**: 144–8.

39 Barker DJP, Morris J, Nelson M. Vegetable consumption and acute appendicitis in 59 areas in England and Wales. *BMJ* 1986;**292**:927–30.

40 Morris J, Barker DJP, Nelson M. Diet, infection and acute appendicitis in Britain and Ireland. *J Epidemiol Community Health* 1987;**41**:44–9.

41 Backett EM. Social patterns of antibody to poliovirus. *Lancet* 1957;**i**:778–83.

42 *Ministry of Health Report of the Committee of Inquiry into the anti-tuberculosis service in Wales and Monmouthshire.* London: HMSO, 1939.

43 Coggon D, Barker DJP, Cruddas M, Oliver RHP. Housing and appendicitis in Anglesey. *J Epidemiol Community Health* 1991;**45**:244–6.

44 Paget Sir J. On a form of chronic inflammation of bones (osteitis deformans). *Medico-Chirurgical Transactions of London* 1877;**60**:37–64.

45 Schmorl G. Ueber osteitis deformans Paget. *Arch Pathol Anat* 1932;**283**:694–751.

46 Pygott F. Paget's disease of bone: the radiological incidence. *Lancet* 1957;**ii**:1170–1.

47 Barker DJP. The epidemiology of Paget's disease of bone. *Br Med Bull* 1984;**40**: 396–400.

48 Barry HC. *Paget's disease of bone.* Edinburgh: Livingstone, 1969.

49 Detheridge FM, Guyer PB, Barker DJP. European distribution of Paget's disease of bone. *BMJ* 1982;**285**:1005–8.

50 Falch JA. Paget's disease in Norway. *Lancet* 1979;**ii**:1022.

51 Barker DJP, Chamberlain AT, Guyer PB, Gardner MJ. Paget's disease of bone: the Lancashire focus. *BMJ* 1980;**280**:1105–7.

52 Piga AM, López-Abente G, Ibáñez AE, Vadillo AG, Lanza MG, Jodra VM. Risk factors for Paget's disease: a new hypothesis. *Int J Epidemiol* 1988;**17**:198–201.

53 Guyer PB, Chamberlain AT. Paget's disease of bone in two American cities *BMJ* 1980; **280**:985.

54 Rosenbaum HD, Hanson DJ. Geographic variation in the prevalence of Paget's disease of bone. *Radiology* 1969;**92**:959–63.

55 Van Meedervoort E, Richter G. Paget's disease of bone in South African blacks. *S Afr Med J* 1976;**50**:1897–9.

56 Guyer PB, Chamberlain AT. Paget's disease of bone in South Africa. *Clin Radiol* 1988;**39**:51–2.

57 Gardner MJ, Guyer PB, Barker DJP. Radiological prevelance of Paget's disease of bone in British migrants to Australia. *BMJ* 1978;**i**:1655–7.

58 Sofaer JA, Holloway SM, Emery AEH. A family study of Paget's disease of bone. *J Epidemiol Community Health* 1983;**37**:226–31.

59 McKusick VA. Mendelian inheritance in man. *Catalogs of autosomal dominant, autosomal recessive and X-linked phenotypes*, 5th ed. Baltimore: Johns Hopkins University Press, 1978:294–5.

60 Rebel A, Basle M, Pouplard A, Kouyoumdjian S, Filmon R, Lepatezour A. Viral antigens in osteoclasts from Paget's disease of bone. *Lancet* 1980;**ii**:344–6.

61 Singer FR, Mills BG. The etiology of Paget's disease of bone. *Clin Orthop* 1977;**127**: 37–42.

62 Barker DJP, Gardner MJ. Distribution of Paget's disease in England, Wales and Scotland and a possible relationship with vitamin D deficiency in childhood. *British J Prev Soc Med* 1974;**28**:226–32.

63 O'Driscoll JB, Anderson DC. Past pets and Paget's disease. *Lancet* 1985;**ii**:919–21.

64 Barker DJP, Detheridge FM. Dogs and Paget's disease. *Lancet* 1985;**ii**:1245.

65 Potts CS. A case of progressive muscular atrophy occurring in a man who had acute poliomyelitis nineteen years previously. *University of Pennsylvania Medical Bulletin* 1903;**16**:31–7.

66 Martyn CN. Poliovirus and motor neuron disease. *J Neurol* 1990;**237**:336–8.

67 Martyn CN, Barker DJP, Osmond C. Motoneuron disease and past poliomyelitis in England and Wales. *Lancet* 1988;**i**:1319–22.

68 Martyn CN, Osmond C. The environment in childhood and risk of motor neurone disease. *J Neurol Neurosurg Psychiatry* 1992;**55**:997–1001.

69 Acheson ED. The epidemiology of multiple sclerosis. In: Mathews WB, ed., *McAlpine's multiple sclerosis*. Edinburgh: Churchill Livingstone, 1985.

70 Lenman JAR, Peters TJ. Herpes zoster and multiple sclerosis. *BMJ* 1969;**2**:218–20.

71 Norrby E. Viral antibodies in multiple sclerosis. *Progress in Medicine and Virology* 1978; **24**:1–39.

72 Martin JR. Herpes simplex virus types 1 and 2 and multiple sclerosis. *Lancet* 1981;**ii**: 777–81.

73 Gay D, Dick G, Upton G. Multiple sclerosis associated with sinusitis: case-controlled study in general practice. *Lancet* 1986;**i**:815–19.

74 Alter M, Cendrowski W. Multiple sclerosis and childhood infections. *Neurology* 1976; **26**:201–4.

75 Operskalski EA, Visscher BR, Malmgren RM, Detels R. A case-control study of multiple sclerosis. *Neurology* 1989;**39**:825–9.

76 Martyn CN, Cruddas M, Compston DAS. Symptomatic Epstein–Barr virus infection and multiple sclerosis. *J Neurol Neurosurg Psychiatry* 1993;**56**:167–8.

9: The undernourished baby

Although the growth of a fetus is influenced by its genes, studies in humans and animals suggest that it is usually limited by the nutrients and oxygen it receives.[1 2] The mother seems to exert a stronger effect on fetal growth than the father. Among half siblings, related only through one parent, those with the same mother have similar birthweights, the correlation coefficient being 0·58. The birthweights of half siblings with the same father are, however, dissimilar, the correlation coefficient being only 0·1.[3] Other studies of relatives have shown that first cousins related through the mother tend to have similar birthweights whereas paternal first cousins do not.[4] Penrose[5] analysed the birthweights of relatives and concluded that 62% of the variation between individuals was the result of the intrauterine environment, 20% was the result of maternal genes and 18% of fetal genes. These and other findings, together with studies in domestic animals, suggest that birth size is controlled by the mother rather than the genetic inheritance from both parents.[6-9]

Maternal–fetal conflict

Haig and others have suggested that the relation between mother and fetus can usefully be viewed as genetic conflict.[10 11] The effects of natural selection on genes expressed in fetuses may be opposed by the effects of natural selection on genes expressed in mothers. Fetal genes will be selected to increase the transfer of nutrients to the fetus so that it grows larger. Maternal genes will be selected to limit transfer to the fetus to protect the mother, and to ensure her survival and that of her children, born and unborn. What is best for the fetus need not be best for its mother, or so it seems.

The theory of parent–child conflict proposes that children are selected to demand more resources from parents than parents are selected to give. Three sets of genes have different interests: the mother's genes, the fetus's genes derived from the mother, and the fetus's genes derived from the father. If the genes of the fetus make excessive demands on the mother, it will prejudice the mother's ability to pass her genes on to other offspring. It is argued that genes derived from the father have been selected to take more resources from the mother's tissues than the genes derived from the mother.[12] The conflict between the maternal and paternal genomes over the nutritional demands that the fetus imposes on its mother may explain why genes derived from one parent can "imprint", or override, the expression of those derived from the other. An example of "genomic imprinting" is that of the genes for insulin-like growth factor II. In the mouse, only those derived from the father are expressed.[13][14]

Maternal constraint of fetal growth

In Walton and Hammond's[15] well known experiments, in which Shetland and Shire horses were crossed, the foals were smaller at birth when the Shetland pony was the mother than when the Shire horse was the mother. As the genetic composition of the two crosses was similar, this implied that the Shetland mother had constrained the growth of the fetus. Similar results were obtained when South Devon cattle, the largest breed of cattle in the British Isles, were crossed with Dexter cattle, the smallest breed.[16] The results of these cross breeding experiments are supported by recent embryo transfer experiments. The size at birth of animal embryos removed from their mothers' uteri is related to the size of the uterus into which they are transferred.[17]

The Ounsteds[18] examined a group of mothers who had growth retarded babies. They found that the mothers were similar in height and other characteristics to a group of controls. Their earlier children, however, had lower mean birthweight. This suggested that these mothers had constrained the intrauterine growth of all their children. Further studies showed that the mothers themselves had had low mean birthweight.

Other studies have shown that the birthweights of mothers are related to those of their children and even their children's children.[19-23] This has led to the conclusion that mothers constrain fetal growth and that the degree of constraint they exert is set when they themselves are *in utero*.[24] Hence sisters, who experience a common level of constraint *in utero*, exert a similar level of constraint on their own fetuses. Although low birthweight is a feature of the families of mothers who have growth retarded babies, it is not a feature of the families of the fathers. Studies of babies who are unusually large at birth have, however, shown that large birthweight is common in the families of both parents. One interpretation of this is that the father influences the fetal growth trajectory only when maternal constraint is relaxed.[24]

The Dutch Hunger Winter has shown how maternal constraint passes from one generation to another. The famine occurred in the western part of the Netherlands during the Second World War.[25] It began in October 1944 after the German occupation forces imposed an embargo on all transport and food supplies—a reprisal for a general rail strike. It ended suddenly, in May 1945, when the Allied armies liberated the Netherlands.

An account of the famine, written immediately after liberation, stated that "the average food intake from all sources, including extra-legal, in October 1944 was approximately 1600 calories. This was reduced to 1300 calories or less in April 1945". Dutch women who were born in Amsterdam during and after the famine, and who experienced famine during the first and second trimesters of their intrauterine lives, have been followed up. Although they themselves had normal birthweight the mean birthweight of their own babies was reduced.[26]

"Maternal constraint" is thought to reflect the limited capacity of the mother to deliver nutrients to her fetus.[27] The amount of nutrients which reaches the fetus reflects the mother's nutrient stores, what she eats during pregnancy, and the processes of digestion, absorption and transport in the blood, and transfer across the placenta. Mothers' height is related to birthweight, so that short women have small babies.[7] Teleologically this form of constraint can be viewed as a way of ensuring that the fetus cannot outgrow the size of the mother's pelvis and birth canal. Mother's pelvic size is not, however, related to the long term changes in the physiology and metabolism of the fetus described in this book. Discussion of maternal constraint in this chapter will therefore focus on influences that determine delivery of nutrients to the fetus.

Fetal adaptation to undernutrition

In common with other living things the growth of the human fetus is plastic. Its major adaptation to undernutrition is to slow its rate of growth. This enhances its ability to survive by reducing the use of substrates and lowering the metabolic rate. It is associated with a redistribution of blood flow to preserve the flow to those tissues that are important for survival, including the brain.[28 29] Though this ensures immediate survival it may be at the price of long term changes which cause disease and reduce survival in the post-reproductive period. Undernutrition in late gestation, for example, may lead to reduced growth of the kidney which develops rapidly at that time. Reduced replication of kidney cells may permanently reduce cell numbers, because after birth there seems to be no capacity for renal cell division to "catch up".[30 31] Whether this reduced number of cells has long term effects may depend on whether the system is stressed, for example, by high salt intake and thereby becomes unable to maintain the volume and composition of body fluids.

At some point before birth the human fetus "sets" its growth trajectory to match the nutrient supply. Thereafter, growth becomes homoeostatically controlled, and largely independent of day to day variation in the availability of nutrients. Growth rates therefore "track" (see chapter 2). This is an example of how adaptations to the early nutritional environment have permanent effects. If this environment changes in later life, through famine, a time of plenty, or migration, people may be disadapted. Perhaps a person who was undernourished as a baby and became a thin short adult, an almost universal experience in China, more readily becomes obese in times of plenty.

The nutrient supply, to which the fetus adapts, depends not only on the nutrient quality of maternal blood, but on other mechanisms including delivery of blood to the fetus. The similarity of birthweight between successive generations of women suggests that the mother's physiological capacity to nourish her fetus is established when she herself is *in utero*. Hence a fetus adapts not only to its mother, but to the environment which its grandmother provided for its mother. Sensitivity to more than one generation allows the fetus to adapt to the environment which has prevailed over many years, rather than only to that at the time of its conception. This might be important in places where there is periodic famine.

Maternal nutrition and birth size

During the last 50 years numerous studies have examined whether the quality of the diet eaten by a pregnant woman influences the size of the baby at birth. The results have been various and contradictory.[32] In retrospect this is unsurprising because we now know that the effects of diet interact with the mother's physiology and metabolism, which determine transport of nutrients to the fetus. One aspect of maternal metabolism which has been intensively studied is how body weight before and during pregnancy relates to birth size.

WEIGHT BEFORE PREGNANCY

Fig 9.1 illustrates the remarkable variety of body form among young women in an affluent country. Whereas in Western countries women like the one in the middle are slim by choice, around the world most women with low body weight in relation to their height have been chronically undernourished since childhood. Women who have low body weight before pregnancy tend to have small babies.[33-35] Chronic undernutrition also influences birthweight through its effect on maternal stature, independent of body weight.[7 36] It may be associated with deficiencies in specific nutrients which influence fetal growth, including vitamins A, C, and D, folate, iron, and zinc. In animals nutrient deficiencies before and immediately after mating lead to reduced head size and length at birth.[37]

Among chronically undernourished mothers high weight gain during pregnancy partly offsets the effects of low weight before pregnancy, although the babies' weights tend to remain below average.[38 39] Observations on obese women point to the importance of pre-pregnant weight in determining

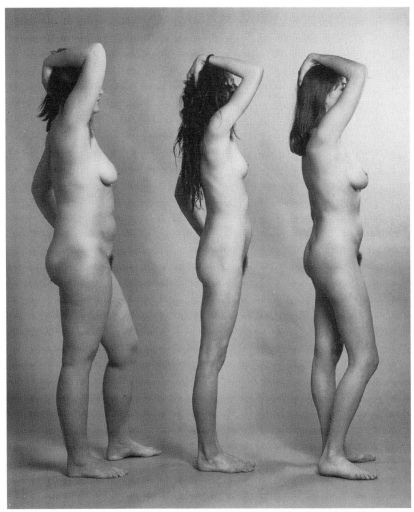

FIG 9.1—*Variations in body fat in normal young women. (Courtesy of the photographer, Helen Garnett.)*

birthweight. Those who gain little weight during pregnancy, or even lose weight, have babies of average or above average weight.[38-42] Among the ways in which the mother's body fat may influence the baby's growth is through differences in protein metabolism. Obese people may conserve protein more efficiently. During starvation they obtain less of their energy from protein breakdown.[43]

The young women in fig 9.1 differ not only in their body weight but in their distribution of body fat. They differ considerably in the relative

125

thickness of their skinfolds at different sites, including the upper arm (triceps), below the shoulder (subscapular), and above the hip (suprailiac). They also have varying amounts of abdominal fat shown by the relative circumference of their waists in relation to their hips. The woman on the left has the highest "waist : hip" ratio. Differences in the proportions of fat in different parts of the body are known to be linked to differences in metabolism. Deposition of fat on the abdomen, for example, is associated with resistance to insulin and an altered balance of sex hormones.[44] The effect of such metabolic differences on the fetus is largely unknown. The possible importance of body fat distribution to the long term health of the baby is, however, shown by recent findings in Jamaica, where the children of mothers with thinner triceps skinfolds had raised blood pressure.[45]

Patterns of fat deposition in adult life may be partly determined by intrauterine growth. A study of men aged 50–70 years showed that lower birthweight, and a higher placental weight : birthweight ratio, were associated with a high waist : hip ratio, independent of total body weight.[46] Similarly, among young men and women in Texas, those with lower birthweights tended to store fat on the trunk, having a high subscapular : triceps skinfold thickness ratio.[47] The tendency to store fat abdominally or on the trunk may be a persisting response to undernutrition and growth failure in fetal life and infancy.

WEIGHT DURING PREGNANCY

The effects on the fetus of low maternal weight gain during pregnancy have been dramatically demonstrated by war-time famines in previously well nourished populations. The Dutch Hunger Winter lasted for seven months and affected women at different stages of pregnancy. Babies exposed to the famine during the first half of gestation, who were born after the famine was lifted, had normal birthweight. Those exposed during the second half of gestation had low birthweight, being 327 g lighter than babies born before the famine.[48][49] The effect of the famine in Wuppertal, Germany, during 1945–46 was less. Calorie intake was reduced to around 2400 a day and birthweight was reduced by around 185 g.[50] The exceptionally severe famine in Leningrad (now St Petersburg) during 1941–43 led to a 530 g fall in mean birthweight.[51] The German blockade of Leningrad between September 1941 and January 1944 prevented supplies from reaching the city for 900 days. During the siege approximately 1 million Leningrad citizens died from a total population of 2·4 million. Most of these deaths occurred during the "hunger winter" of November 1941 to February 1942 when the siege was in full force and the average daily ration was about 300 calories, composed almost entirely of carbohydrate. Nearly 50% of all term infants exposed to famine during the second half of gestation weighed less than 2500 g.

In Western countries lesser degrees of undernutrition during pregnancy, reflected in low maternal weight gain, are common. They lead to modest reductions in birthweight.[52-55] The weak relationship between maternal weight gain in pregnancy and birth size has contributed to the myth that, in affluent populations, nutrition has little effect on fetal growth.[56] The relationship between calorie intake in pregnancy and birthweight, found in observational studies and trials, is of varying size and generally less than had been expected.[57] In one of the best known studies the diets of primagravid women were recorded by weighed food intakes and food diaries during the seventh month of pregnancy.[58] Calorie intake was associated with birthweight in that women who consumed less than 1800 calories per day had babies who weighed 240 g less than those of mothers who ate 3000 and more calories. However, women who were heavier at 30 weeks had larger babies and, after allowing for this, the correlation with calorie intake disappeared.

In some trials supplementation of the mother's diet has led to an increase in mean birthweight, though generally of small size. One trial of protein–calorie supplementation, among poorly nourished mothers in New York City, produced a fall in mean birthweight.[59] This unexpected result led to a re-analysis of all reported supplementation trials:[60] supplements with a low percentage of calories as protein were found to have increased birthweight whereas supplements with a high protein density reduced birthweight.

A number of studies support the idea that the inconsistency in the results of different trials could be the result of differing effects in women whose nutritional states differed. Underweight women with high calorie intakes during pregnancy have babies of similar size to those of overweight women with low calorie intakes. A trial among Asian women living in England suggested that the babies of women whose triceps skinfold thickness did not increase in mid-pregnancy benefited most from protein and energy supplementation.[61] In The Gambia, energy supplementation increased birthweight only during the wet season, a time when food is scarce and women work hard planting crops.[62] In the New York study only the babies of mothers who smoked cigarettes benefited;[59] it is not known whether this reflected the different diets of smokers and non-smokers.

In summary the evidence suggests that it is not merely the mother's diet during pregnancy, but her nutritional experience over many years, which controls the growth of the fetus. Her own fetal life will have influenced her ability to sustain the growth of her baby. McCarrison[63] wrote in 1937 "the satisfaction of nutritional needs in pregnancy begins with the antenatal lives of the mothers of our race. It must continue during the period of their growth and development up to, during and following the period when they find their fulfilment in motherhood".

Maternal nutrition, body proportions at birth and infant growth

Chapters 3–6 showed that physiological disorders in adult life are linked not only to birthweight but to body proportions at birth. Babies who are thin at birth (see fig 3.8 in chapter 3) develop different disorders from babies who are short (see fig 3.9 in chapter 3). This is consistent with animal studies which show that fetal undernutrition may lead to newborns with similar overall body size but marked differences in the proportional size of different organs (see chapter 2).

There is limited information about the maternal influences that determine different body proportions at birth. Babies exposed to the Dutch Hunger Winter during the last trimester had a disproportionate reduction in birth-weight in relation to length.[25][49] Other studies have shown reduced protein intake during pregnancy to be associated with shortness at birth.[64] The consensus of evidence is that, if the blood supply to the fetus is restricted, it leads to reduced body length although the head and brain are spared.[8] Animal experiments show that the effects of undernutrition, whether through low nutrient intake or inadequate blood flow, depend on its timing and duration (see page 18). Undernutrition in mid or late gestation is associated with disproportionate growth, reflected in thinness or shortness at birth. Chronic nutritional deprivation sustained from early pregnancy is associated with symmetrical growth failure in head size and length.[8]

An important difference between fetal growth in the developing countries and that in Western countries is that symmetrical growth retardation (fig 9.2) is common in developing countries whereas disproportionate, or "asymmetrical", growth retardation prevails in Western countries.[8] Babies with symmetrical growth retardation may be more prone to neurodevelopmental impairment, whereas those with asymmetrical growth retardation may be more at risk of perinatal death.[65][66]

The pattern of infant growth which follows reduced intrauterine growth differs according to the body proportions at birth.[66][67] Thin babies tend to catch up in weight during infancy whereas disproportionately short and symmetrically small babies do not. Among men the stronger relationship of coronary heart disease to weight at one year than to birthweight (see chapter 3) is thought to reflect an association with disproportionate short-ness at birth and consequent failure of infant growth.

Maternal nutrition and the placenta

The fetus can become undernourished in spite of an adequate nutrient supply from the mother if transport across the placenta is inadequate. This may result from poor implantation or breakdown of feedback control between the fetus and placenta. If nutrient supply to the placenta is reduced,

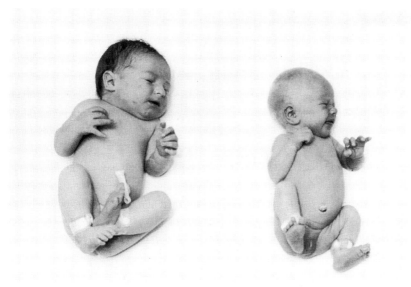

FIG 9.2—*The newborn baby on the right is symmetrically smaller than the baby on the left.*

not only is fetal growth suppressed but also the placenta mediates secondary changes in maternal metabolism and cardiovascular function. In some circumstances the placenta may adapt to reduced nutrient supply from the mother by enlarging.

Although birthweight and placental weight are highly correlated, placental weight predicts adult disorders independent of birthweight. Babies with a placenta that is disproportionately large in relation to their birthweight are at increased risk of death from cardiovascular disease,[68] raised blood pressure,[69 70] impaired glucose tolerance,[71] and raised plasma fibrinogen concentrations.[72] The strength of these associations is illustrated in table 4.6 in chapter 4 (page 60).

Some animal studies have shown that maternal undernutrition in early/mid-pregnancy reduces placental weight.[73 74] Other studies show that undernutrition in mid-pregnancy increases placental weight, but the findings are not readily reproducible.[75-77] McCrabb suggested that this might be the result of different maternal nutritional reserves before conception.[77] Subsequently Robinson and colleagues in Adelaide showed that good nutrition around the time of conception, followed by a restricted diet in mid-pregnancy, stimulated placental growth in sheep.[78] These observations on the effect of a changing plane of nutrition during pregnancy are consistent

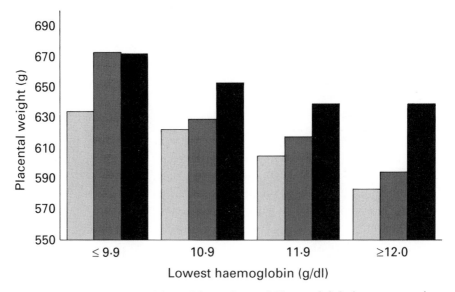

FIG 9.3—*Mean placental weight and lowest haemoglobin recorded during pregnancy in 8684 women in Oxford delivered during 1987–89. Fall in mean corpuscular volume (fl):* □*<4;* ▦*4–6;* ■*>6.*

with empirical practices in sheep farming, whereby ewes are moved to poorer pasture for some weeks after mating.

In humans, Beischer's study in five countries has shown that anaemia during pregnancy is associated with increased placental size at birth.[79] Mild hypoxaemia associated with high altitude has the same association, and Clapp and colleagues have demonstrated that physical exercise by the mother in mid-gestation is associated with increased placental volume.[80–82] Fig 9.3 is taken from a study of 8684 pregnant women in Oxford.[83] Those whose haemoglobin concentration fell to lower values during pregnancy had larger placentas. Subsequent studies showed that, among women with low haemoglobin, placental volume was already increased at 18 weeks of pregnancy.[84] Furthermore, Wheeler and colleagues showed that maternal haemoglobin concentrations between nine and 11 weeks of pregnancy were inversely related to the maternal serum concentrations of chorionic gonadotrophin and placental lactogen, hormones synthesised by the placenta.[85] Maternal serum ferritin concentrations were not related to these two hormones. The association with haemoglobin was not explained by the effects of haemodilution and is thought to reflect the effects of the oxygen content of maternal blood on placental development and function. Hypoxia may stimulate blood vessel formation in the growing placenta.

Long term effects of fetal undernutrition

The fetus's major physiological adaptation to undernutrition is to restrict its growth (see page 123). This enhances its ability to survive by reducing the use of substrates and lowering the metabolic rate. Harding's data, shown in fig 2.4, illustrate how the fetus's ability to adapt to undernutrition depends on its previous growth rate, more rapidly growing fetuses being less able to adapt.[86 87] The long term consequences of reduced fetal growth described in previous chapters raise a number of questions. What are the influences that alter fetal growth? How does the fetus respond? How are the long term cardiovascular, metabolic, and endocrine consequences programmed? Knowledge is still scanty, but it is possible to set out a broad framework within which these questions can be explored.

EARLY PREGNANCY

The concentrations of nutrients in the earliest stages of pregnancy influence growth of the embryo. Animal studies have shown that birth size can be profoundly changed by a brief period of in vitro culture before implantation. Suboptimal nutrition before implantation retards growth and development, the one-cell embryo being particularly sensitive. The early embryo is selective in its use of nutrients and respires pyruvate, lactate, and amino acids such as glutamine rather than glucose.[88] Before implantation it switches to glucose based metabolism, and low glucose concentrations retard its growth and development.[89] Paradoxically, perhaps, high glucose concentrations, which accompany maternal diabetes, also delay embryonic growth. This effect contrasts with the accelerated growth associated with high glucose concentrations in late pregnancy. The baby which is undernourished from an early stage of gestation tends to be proportionately small at birth (see fig 9.2). Early down-regulation of its growth may protect it from undernutrition in late gestation.

MID-PREGNANCY

The placenta grows faster than the fetus in mid-pregnancy. Nutrient deficiency may therefore affect fetal growth by changing the interaction between the fetus and the placenta. Although severe maternal undernutrition restricts growth of fetus and placenta, mild undernutrition may lead to increased placental but not fetal size.[76] This placental overgrowth may be an adaptation to sustain nutrient supply from the mother. Localised placental hypertrophy can also be induced experimentally in sheep by reducing the number of implantation sites. Owens and Robinson[90] have shown that the compensatory growth at the remaining sites occurs before there is noticeable retardation of fetal growth, and may be a sensitive, early response to reduced nutrient supply.

During undernutrition fetal growth may be sacrificed to maintain placental function. In animals oxygen, glucose, and amino acids may be redistributed, so that the placenta reduces its consumption of oxygen and glucose while maintaining a large output of lactate to the fetus.[91] The lactate is partly derived from amino acids of fetal origin, and the fetus may waste and be thin at birth.[92] There is evidence for similar metabolic changes in growth retarded human fetuses, in whom wasting has been observed using ultrasonography.[93-95]

LATE PREGNANCY

In late gestation undernutrition results in immediate slowing of fetal growth. Acute undernutrition causes prompt slowing of fetal growth associated with fetal catabolism,[87] but fetal growth rapidly resumes when nutrition is restored. In contrast, prolonged undernutrition may irreversibly slow the rate of fetal growth in lambs and lead to reduced length at birth.[96] The basis of this irreversibility is uncertain, but it is reflected in the clinical observation that children with intrauterine growth retardation who show postnatal growth failure are those with evidence of more prolonged intrauterine growth retardation.[97]

SUMMARY

Undernutrition changes the pattern of fetal and placental growth. In early pregnancy it retards embryonic growth and may result in proportionately small babies (see fig 9.2). Undernutrition in mid-pregnancy may change the interactions between fetus and placenta. The placenta may be either small or hypertrophied, and the fetus may waste (see fig 3.8 in chapter 3) as amino acids are diverted to the placenta for energy production. Prolonged undernutrition in late gestation leads to shortness at birth (see fig 3.9).

Hormonal responses to fetal undernutrition

Responses to undernutrition *in utero* include changes in the concentrations of fetal and placental hormones which control growth (chapter 2). Fetal insulin and the insulin-like growth factors (IGFs) are thought to have a central role in the regulation of growth, responding rapidly to changes in nutrition.[98] If a mother decreases her food intake fetal insulin, IGF and glucose concentrations fall (possibly through the effect of decreased maternal IGF). This leads to reduced transfer of amino acids and glucose from mother to fetus, and reduced rates of fetal growth.[99] In late gestation and after birth the fetus's growth hormone and IGF axis take over, from insulin, a central role in driving linear growth.

Following undernutrition persistent changes in the production of the hormones that control growth, or in the sensitivity of tissues to them, could permanently program metabolism.[100 101] For example, the fetus may acquire a persisting deficiency in insulin production or may become resistant to insulin. After birth insulin deficiency and resistance would be manifest through effects on glucose metabolism: as described in chapter 6, non-insulin dependent diabetes may originate in this way. Babies who are thin at birth are now known to be insulin resistant as adults and to have increased death rates from cardiovascular disease.

Gluckman proposed that babies who are short at birth and grow slowly in infancy may have persisting defects in their growth hormone and IGF axes which suggest either growth hormone deficiency or resistance.[101-7] The Hertfordshire and Sheffield studies have shown that babies who are short at birth, with a small liver, as measured by the abdominal circumference, and who fail to gain weight in infancy, have raised plasma concentrations of low density lipoprotein cholesterol and plasma fibrinogen as adults (chapter 5) and raised death rates from coronary heart disease (chapter 3). Adults with growth hormone deficiency have an increased mortality from cardiovascular disease, lower serum high density lipoprotein and raised triglyceride concentrations, increased body mass, and raised blood pressure.[108 109] Administration of growth hormone to normal subjects stimulates the low density lipoprotein cholesterol receptor in the liver and lowers serum cholesterol concentrations by 25%.[110]

A framework of ideas

Fig 9.4 gives a framework within which the links between fetal undernutrition and cardiovascular disease can be explored. It is a working hypothesis and will need to be re-evaluated as more information becomes available.

Undernutrition in early gestation leads to a baby who is symmetrically small at birth (see fig 9.2), and remains small in infancy. As yet, little is known about their adult disorders but, as this type of growth retardation is common in areas of the less developed world including China, one may speculate that it predisposes to hypertension and haemorrhagic stroke but not to coronary heart disease.

Undernutrition in mid-gestation leads to a thin baby (see fig 3.8) whose growth catches up during infancy. As an adult he or she is insulin resistant

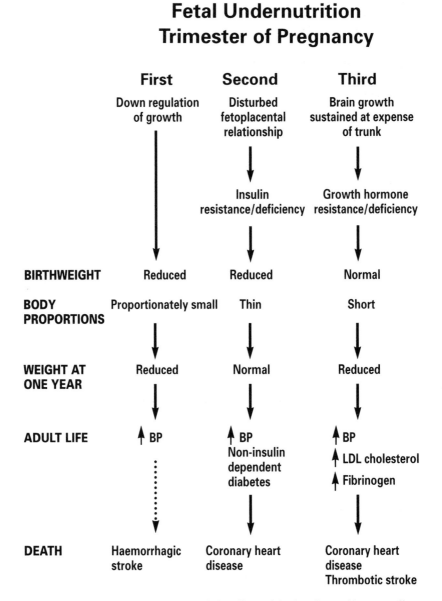

Fetal Undernutrition
Trimester of Pregnancy

	First	**Second**	**Third**
	Down regulation of growth	Disturbed fetoplacental relationship	Brain growth sustained at expense of trunk
		Insulin resistance/deficiency	Growth hormone resistance/deficiency
BIRTHWEIGHT	Reduced	Reduced	Normal
BODY PROPORTIONS	Proportionately small	Thin	Short
WEIGHT AT ONE YEAR	Reduced	Normal	Reduced
ADULT LIFE	↑ BP	↑ BP Non-insulin dependent diabetes	↑ BP ↑ LDL cholesterol ↑ Fibrinogen
DEATH	Haemorrhagic stroke	Coronary heart disease	Coronary heart disease Thrombotic stroke

FIG 9.4—*Diagrammatic representation of the effects of fetal undernutrition according to trimester of pregnancy.*

and is predisposed to non-insulin dependent diabetes, hypertension, and coronary heart disease.

Undernutrition in late gestation leads to a baby that is relatively short in relation to its head size (see fig 3.9), which may have a normal birthweight but grows slowly during infancy. It may be deficient in growth hormone or resistant. As an adult he or she has raised blood cholesterol and fibrinogen concentrations, and is predisposed to coronary heart disease and stroke.

Summary

The growth of a baby is constrained by the nutrients and oxygen it receives from its mother. A mother's ability to nourish her baby is established during her own fetal life and by her nutritional experience over many years before pregnancy. The baby's major adaptation to undernutrition is to reduce its growth rate although in some circumstances the placenta may enlarge. Slowing of growth is associated with changes in the production of fetal hormones, including insulin and growth hormone, and the sensitivity of tissues to them. Persistence of these changes, together with changes in the structure of organs, and the types and number of cells within them, may permanently program the body's metabolism.

1 McCance RA, Widdowson EM. The determinants of growth and form. *Proc R Soc Lond [Biol]* 1974;**185**:1–17.
2 Gluckman PD, Breier BH, Oliver M, Harding JE, Bassett NS. Fetal growth in late gestation—A constrained pattern of growth. *Acta Paediatr Scand Suppl* 1990;**367**: 105–10.
3 Morton NE. The inheritance of human birth weight. *Ann Hum Genet* 1955;**20**:123–34.
4 Robson EB. Birth weight in cousins. *Ann Hum Genet* 1955;**19**:262–8.
5 Penrose LS. Some recent trends in human genetics. *Caryologia* 1954;**6**(suppl):521–9.
6 Lush JL, Hetzer HO, Culbertson CC. Factors affecting birth weights of swine. *Genetics* 1934;**19**:329–43.
7 Cawley RH, McKeown T, Record RG. Parental stature and birth weight. *Ann Hum Genet* 1954;**6**:448–56.
8 Kline J, Stein Z, Susser M. *Conception to birth—epidemiology of prenatal development.* New York: Oxford University Press, 1976.
9 Roberts DF. The genetics of human growth. In: Falkner F, Tanner JM, eds, *Human growth*, vol 3, *Methodology: ecological, genetic and nutritional effects on growth*. New York: Plenum Press, 1986.
10 Trivers RL. Parent-offspring conflict. *Am Zool* 1974;**14**:249–64.
11 Moore T, Haig D. Genomic imprinting in mammalian development: a prenatal tug of war. *Trends Genet* 1991;**7**:45–9.
12 Haig D, Graham C. Genomic imprinting and the strange case of the insulin-like growth factor II receptor. *Cell* 1991;**64**:1045–6.
13 Hall JG. Genomic imprinting: review and relevance to human diseases. *Am J Hum Genet* 1990;**46**:857–73.
14 De Chiara TM, Robertson EJ, Efstratiadis A. Parental imprinting of the mouse insulin-like growth factor II gene. *Cell* 1991;**64**:849–59.
15 Walton A, Hammond J. The maternal effects on growth and conformation in Shire horse-Shetland pony crosses. *Proc R Soc Lond [Biol]* 1938;**125**:311–35.

16 Joubert DM, Hammond J. A crossbreeding experiment with cattle with special reference to the maternal effect in South Devon-Dexter crosses. *J Agric Sci* 1958;**51**: 325–41.

17 Snow MHL. Effects of genome on size at birth. In: Sharp F, Fraser RB, Milner RDG, eds, *Fetal growth*. London: Royal College of Obstetricians and Gynaecologists, 1989; 3–12.

18 Ounsted M, Ounsted C. Maternal regulation of intra-uterine growth. *Nature* 1966;**212**: 995–7.

19 Hackman E, Emanuel I, Van Bolle G, Daling J. Maternal birth weight and subsequent pregnancy outcome. *JAMA* 1983;**250**:2016–19.

20 Klebanoff MA, Graubard B, Kessel SS, Berendes HW. Low birth weight across generations. *JAMA* 1984;**252**:2423–7.

21 Carr-Hill R, Campbell DM, Hall MH, Meredith A. Is birth weight determined genetically? *BMJ* 1987;**295**:687–9.

22 Alberman E, Emanuel I, Filarkti H, Evans SJW. The contrasting effects of parental birthweight and gestational age on the birthweight of offspring. *Pediatric and Perinatal Epidemiology* 1992;**6**:134–44.

23 Emanuel I, Filkarti H, Alberman E, Evans SJW. Intergenerational studies of human birthweight from the 1958 birth cohort. I. Evidence for a multigenerational effect. *Br J Obstet Gynaecol* 1992;**99**:67–74.

24 Ounsted M, Scott A, Ounsted C. Transmission through the female line of a mechanism constraining human fetal growth. *Ann Hum Biol* 1986;**13**:143–51.

25 Stein ZA, Susser MW. The Dutch Famine, 1944–45, and the reproductive process. I. Effects on six indices at birth. *Pediatr Res* 1975;**9**:70–6.

26 Lumey LH. Decreased birthweights in infants after maternal in utero exposure to the Dutch famine of 1944–45. *Paediatric and Perinatal Epidemiology* 1992;**6**:240–53.

27 Gluckman P, Harding J. The regulation of fetal growth. In: Hernandez M, Argente J, eds, *Human growth: basic and clinical aspects*. Elsevier, Amsterdam, 1992:253–9.

28 Campbell AGM, Dawes GS, Fishman AP, Hyman AI. Regional redistribution of blood flow in the mature fetal lamb. *Circulation Research* 1967;**21**:229–35.

29 Rudolph AM. The fetal circulation and its response to stress. *J Dev Physiol* 1984;**6**: 11–19.

30 Widdowson EM. Immediate and long-term consequences of being large or small at birth: a comparative approach. In: Elliott K, Knight J, eds, *Size at birth. Ciba Symposium 27*. Amsterdam: Elsevier, 1974:65–82.

31 Hinchliffe SA, Lynch MRJ, Sargent PH, Howard CV, Van Velzen D. The effect of intrauterine growth retardation on the development of renal nephrons. *Br J Obstet Gynecol* 1992;**99**:296–301.

32 Rosso P. *Nutrition and metabolism in pregnancy—mother and fetus*. New York: Oxford University Press, 1990.

33 Tompkins WT, Wiehl DG, Mitchell RMcN. The underweight patient as an increased obstetric hazard. *Am J Obstet Gynecol* 1955;**69**:114–23.

34 Love EJ, Kinch RAH. Factors influencing the birth weight in normal pregnancy. *Am J Obstet Gynecol* 1965;**91**:342–9.

35 Edwards LE, Alton IR, Barrada MI, Hakanson EY. Pregnancy in the underweight woman. Course 'outcome' and growth patterns of the infant. *Am J Obstet Gynecol* 1979;**135**:297–302.

36 Baird D. The influence of social and economic factors on stillbirths and neonatal deaths. *Journal of Obstetrics and Gynaecology of the British Empire* 1945;**52**:339–66.

37 Doyle W, Crawford MA, Wynn AHA, Wynn SW. The association between maternal diet and birth dimensions. *Journal of Nutritional Medicine* 1990;**1**:9–17.

38 Eastman NJ, Jackson E. Weight relationships in pregnancy I. The bearing of maternal weight gain and pre-pregnancy weight on birth weight in full term pregnancies. *Obstet Gynecol Surv* 1968;**23**:1003–24.

39 Rosso P. Nutrition and maternal-fetal exchange. *Am J Clin Nutr* 1981;**34**:744–55.

40 Simpson JW, Lawless RW, Mitchell AC. Responsibility of the obstetrician to the fetus. II. Influence of prepregnancy weight and pregnancy weight gain on birthweight. *Obstet Gynecol* 1975;**45**:481–7.

41 Edwards LE, Dickes WF, Alton IR, Hakanson EY. Pregnancy in the massively obese: course, outcome, and obesity prognosis of the infant. *Am J Obstet Gynecol* 1978;**131**: 479–83.
42 Abrams BF, Laros RK. Prepregnancy weight, weight gain, and birth weight. *Am J Obstet Gynecol* 1986;**154**:503–9.
43 Henry CJK. Quantitative relationships between protein and energy metabolism: influence of body composition. In *Protein-energy interactions*. Switzerland: Nestlé Foundation, 1992:191–200.
44 Björntorp P. Adipose tissue distribution and function. *Int J Obesity* 1991;**15**:67–81.
45 Godfrey KM, Forrester T, Barker DJP *et al.* Maternal nutritional status in pregnancy and blood pressure in childhood. *Br J Obstet Gynaecol* 1994;**101**: in press.
46 Law CM, Barker DJP, Osmond C, Fall CHD, Simmonds SJ. Early growth and abdominal fatness in adult life. *J Epidemiol Community Health* 1992;**46**:184–6.
47 Valdey R, Athens MA, Thompson GH, Bradshaw BS, Stern MP. Birthweight and adult health outcomes in a biethnic U.S. population. *Diabetologia* 1994 in press.
48 Smith CA. The effect of wartime starvation in Holland upon pregnancy and its product. *Am J Obstet Gynecol* 1947;**53**:599–608.
49 Stein Z, Susser M, Saenger G, Marolla F. *Famine and human development: The Dutch Hunger Winter of 1944/45*. New York: Oxford University Press, 1975.
50 Dean RFA. The size of the baby at birth and the yield of breast milk. In: *Studies of undernutrition. Wuppertal 1946–9*. London: HMSO 346–78. (Medical Research Council Special Report Series, No. 275, 1951.)
51 Antonov AN. Children born during the siege of Leningrad in 1942. *J Pediatr* 1947;**30**: 250–9.
52 Susser M. Maternal weight gain, infant birthweight and diet: causal sequences. *Am J Clin Nutr* 1991;**53**:1384–96.
53 Niswander K, Jackson EC. Physical characteristics of the gravida and their association with birth weight and perinatal death. *Am J Obstet Gynecol* 1974;**119**:306–13.
54 Gormican A, Valentine J, Satter E. Relationships of maternal weight gain, prepregnancy weight, and infant birthweight. *J Am Diet Assoc* 1980;**77**:662–7.
55 Hytten FE, Chamberlain G. *Clinical physiology in obstetrics*. Oxford: Blackwell Scientific, 1980.
56 Maternal nutrition and low birth-weight. *Lancet* 1975;**ii**:445.
57 Lechtig A, Klein RE. Pre-natal nutrition and birth weight: is there a causal association? In: J Dobbing, ed., *Maternal nutrition in pregnancy—eating for two?* London: Academic Press, 1981:131–83.
58 Thomson AM. Diet in pregnancy. 3. Diet in relation to the course and outcome of pregnancy. *Br J Nutr* 1959;**13**:509–25.
59 Rush D, Stein Z, Susser M. A randomized controlled trial of prenatal nutritional supplementation in New York City. *Pediatrics* 1980;**65**:683–97.
60 Rush D. Effects of changes in maternal energy and protein intake during pregnancy, with special reference to fetal growth. In: Sharp F, Fraser RB, Milner RDG, eds, *Fetal growth*. London: Springer Verlag, 1989:203–29.
61 Viegas OAC, Scott PH, Cole TJ, Needham PG, Wharton BA. Dietary protein energy supplementation of pregnant Asian mothers at Sorrento, Birmingham. II: Selective during the third trimester only. *BMJ* 1982;**285**:592–5.
62 Prentice AM, Watkinson M, Whitehead RG, Lamb WH. Prenatal dietary supplementation of African women and birthweight. *Lancet* 1983;**i**:489–91.
63 McCarrison R. Nutritional needs in pregnancy. *BMJ* 1937;**ii**:256–7.
64 Burke BS, Harding VV, Stuart HC. Nutrition studies during pregnancy. IV. Relation of protein content of mother's diet during pregnancy to birth length, birth weight, and condition of infant at birth. *J Pediatr* 1948;**32**:506–15.
65 Walther FJ, Ramaekers LHJ. Neonatal mortality of SGA infants in relation to their nutritional status at birth. *Acta Paediatr Scand* 1982;**71**:437–40.
66 Villar J, Smeriglio V, Martorell R, Brown CH, Klein RE. Heterogeneous growth and mental development of intrauterine growth retarded infants during the first 3 years of life. *Pediatrics* 1984;**74**:783–91.

67 Holmes GE, Miller HC, Hassanein K, Lansky SB, Groggin JE. Postnatal somatic growth in infants with atypical fetal growth patterns. *Am J Dis Child* 1977;**3**: 1078–83.

68 Barker DJP, Osmond C, Simmonds SJ, Wield GA. The relation of small head circumference and thinness at birth to death from cardiovascular disease in adult life. *BMJ* 1993;**306**:422–6.

69 Barker DJP, Bull AR, Osmond C, Simmonds SJ. Fetal and placental size and risk of hypertension in adult life. *BMJ* 1990;**301**:259–62.

70 Law CM, Barker DJP, Bull AR, Osmond C. Maternal and fetal influences on blood pressure. *Arch Dis Child* 1991;**66**:1291–5.

71 Phipps K, Barker DJP, Hales CN, Fall CHD, Osmond C, Clark PMS. Fetal growth and impaired glucose tolerance in men and women. *Diabetologia* 1993;**36**:225–8.

72 Barker DJP, Meade TW, Fall CHD *et al.* Relation of fetal and infant growth to plasma fibrinogen and factor VII concentrations in adult life. *BMJ* 1992;**304**:148–52.

73 Everitt GC. Maternal undernutrition and retarded foetal development in the Merino sheep. *Nature* 1964;**201**:1341–2.

74 Wallace AM. The growth of lambs before and after birth in relation to the level of nutrition. *Journal of Agricultural Science* 1984;**38**:243–302.

75 Faichney GJ, White GA. Effects of maternal nutritional status on fetal and placental growth and on fetal urea synthesis. *Aust J Biol Sci* 1987;**40**:365–77.

76 McCrabb GJ, Egan AR, Hosking BJ. Maternal undernutrition during mid-pregnancy in sheep. Placental size and its relationship to calcium transfer during late pregnancy. *Br J Nutr* 1991;**65**:157–68.

77 McCrabb GJ, Egan AR, Hosking BJ. Maternal undernutrition during mid-pregnancy in sheep: variable effects on placental growth. *Journal of Agricultural Science* 1992; **118**:127–32.

78 DeBarro TM, Owens J, Earl CR, Robinson JS. Nutrition during early/mid pregnancy interacts with mating weight to affect placental weight in sheep. *Australian Society for Reproductive Biology, Adelaide* 1992 (Abstract).

79 Beischer NA, Sivasamboo R, Vohra S, Silpisornkosal S, Reid S. Placental hypertrophy in severe pregnancy anaemia. *Journal of Obstetrics and Gynaecology of the British Commonwealth* 1970;**77**:398–409.

80 Meyer MB. Effects of maternal smoking and altitude on birth weight and gestation. In: Reed DM, Stanley FJ, eds, *The epidemiology of prematurity.* Baltimore: Urban and Schwarzenberg, 1977:81–104.

81 Mayhew TM, Jackson MR, Haas JD. Oxygen diffusive conductances of human placentae from term pregnancies at low and high altitudes. *Placenta* 1990;**11**: 493–503.

82 Clapp JF III, Rizk KH. Effect of recreational exercise on midtrimester placental growth. *Am J Obstet Gynecol* 1992;**167**:1518–21.

83 Godfrey KM, Redman CWG, Barker DJP, Osmond C. The effect of maternal anaemia and iron deficiency on the ratio of fetal weight to placental weight. *Br J Obstet Gynaecol* 1991;**98**:886–91.

84 Howe D, Wheeler T. Maternal iron stores and placental growth. *J Physiol* 1994 (In press).

85 Wheeler T, Sollero C, Alderman S, Landen J, Anthony F, Osmond C. Relation between maternal haemoglobin and placental hormone concentrations in early pregnancy. *Lancet* 1994;**343**:511–13.

86 Widdowson EM, McCance RA. The effect of finite periods of undernutrition at different ages on the composition and subsequent development of the rat. *Proc R Soc Lond [Biol]* 1963; **158**:329–42.

87 Harding JE, Liu L, Evans PC, Oliver M, Gluckman PD. Intrauterine feeding of the growth retarded fetus: can we help? *Early Hum Dev* 1992;**29**:193–7.

88 Leese HJ. The energy metabolism of the pre-implantation embryo. In: *Early embryo development and paracrine relationships.* New York: Alan R Liss, 1990:67–78.

89 Gott AL, Hardy K, Winston RML, Leese HJ. Non-invasive measurement of pyruvate and glucose uptake and lactate production by single human preimplantation embryos. *Hum Reproduction* 1990;**5**:104–8.

90 Owens JA, Robinson JS. The effect of experimental manipulation of placental growth and development. In: Cockburn F, ed. *Fetal and neonatal growth*. Chichester: John Wiley and Sons, 1988:49–77.

91 Owens JA, Falconer J, Robinson JS. Effect of restriction of placental growth on fetal and utero-placental metabolism. *J Dev Physiol* 1987;**9**:225–38.

92 Owens JA. Endocrine and substrate control of fetal growth: placental and maternal influences and insulin-like growth factors. *Reproduction Fertility and Development* 1990;**3**:501–17.

93 Divon MY, Chamberlain PF, Sipos L, Mannind FA, Platt LD. Identification of the small for gestational age fetus with the use of gestational age-independent indices of fetal growth. *Am J Obstet Gynecol* 1986;**155**:1197–201.

94 Soothill PW, Nicolaides KH, Campbell S. Prenatal asphyxia, hyperlacticaemia, hypoglycaemia and erythroblastosis in growth retarded fetuses. *BMJ* 1987;**294**: 1051–6.

95 Cetin I, Corbetta C, Sereni LP *et al*. Umbilical amino acid concentrations in normal growth-retarded fetuses sampled in utero by cordocentesis. *Am J Obstet Gynecol* 1990;**162**:253–61.

96 Mellor DJ, Murray L. Effects on the rate of increase in fetal girth of refeeding ewes after short periods of severe undernutrition during late pregnancy. *Res Vet Sci* 1982; **32**:377–82.

97 Fancourt R, Campbell S, Harvery D, Norman AP. Follow-up study of small-for-dates babies. *BMJ* 1976;**i**:1435–7.

98 Fowden AL. The role of insulin in prenatal growth. *J Dev Physiol* 1989;**12**:173–82.

99 Oliver MH, Harding JE, Breier BH, Evans PC, Gluckman PD. Glucose but not a mixed amino acid infusion regulates plasma insulin-like growth factor (IGF)-I concentrations in fetal sheep. *Pediatr Res* 1993;**34**:62–5.

100 Hales CN, Barker DJP. Type 2 (non-insulin-dependent) diabetes mellitus: the thrifty phenotype hypothesis. *Diabetologia* 1992;**35**:595–601.

101 Barker DJP, Gluckman PD, Godfrey KM, Harding JE, Owens JA, Robinson JS. Fetal nutrition and cardiovascular disease in adult life. *Lancet* 1993;**341**:938–41.

102 Furuhashi N, Fukaya T, Kono H, *et al*. Cord serum growth hormone in the human fetus. Sex difference and a negative correlation with birth weight. *Gynecol Obstet Invest* 1983;**16**:119–24.

103 Thieriot-Prevost G, Boccara JF, Francoual C, Badoual J, Job JC. Serum insulin-like growth factor 1 and serum growth-promoting activity during the first postnatal year in infants with intrauterine growth retardation. *Pediatr Res* 1988;**24**:380–3.

104 Deiber M, Chatelain P, Naville D, Putet G, Salle B. Functional hypersomatotropism in small for gestational age (SGA) newborn infants. *J Clin Endocrinol Metab* 1989;**68**: 232.

105 Job JC, Chatelain P, Rochiccioli P, Ponte C, Oliver M, Sagard L. Growth hormone response to a bolus injection of 1–44 growth-hormone-releasing hormone in very short children with intrauterine onset of growth failure. *Horm Res* 1990;**33**:161–5.

106 Lassarre C, Hardouin S, Daffos F, Forestier F, Frankenne F, Binoux M. Serum insulin-like growth factor and insulin-like growth factor binding proteins in normal subjects and in subjects with intrauterine growth retardation. *Pediatr Res* 1991;**29**: 219–25.

107 Gluckman PD, Gunn AJ, Wray A, *et al*. Congenital idiopathic growth hormone deficiency is associated with prenatal and early postnatal growth failure. *J Pediatr* 1992;**121**:920–3.

108 Rosen T, Bengtsson BA. Premature mortality due to cardiac disease in hypopituitarism. *Lancet* 1990;**336**:285–8.

109 Rosen T, Eden S, Larson G, Wilhelmsen L, Bengtsson B. Cardiovascular risk factors in adult patients with growth hormone deficiency. *Acta Endocrinol* 1993;**129**: 195–200.

110 Rudling M, Norstedt G, Olivecrona H, Reihner E, Gustafsson J-Å, Angelin B. Importance of growth hormone for the induction of hepatic low density lipoprotein receptors. *Proc Nat Acad Sci* 1992;**89**:6983–7.

10: Preventing disease: lessons from the past

The previous chapter outlined the scientific agenda which now has to be explored if we are to understand how the fetus is nourished, and how its nourishment may be improved. It may be some while before understanding progresses to the point where effective advice can be given to women before and during pregnancy. Meanwhile, history gives an insight into the social conditions which have affected the wellbeing of mothers and their babies and, in consequence, may have changed the life expectancy of their children.

Three Lancashire towns[1]

In Lancashire, England, the cotton industry was harsh to mothers and their babies. Fig 10.1 shows women employed in a mill in Preston, who worked during pregnancy and returned soon after delivery:[2]

> Many women returned to full time work just a few days after having had a baby and there was growing concern that this was contributing towards the high infant death rate in Preston. In 1886 Dr James Rigby produced a critical enquiry on the subject. He described a day in the life of a young mother. She would, he said, have to get up at 5.30am, wrap the baby in a shawl and take it to a nurse who would care for it during the day. These baby-minders had little concern for the children in their care and often drugged them heavily. At 8.30 the mother would rush back from the mill to breast feed her baby and would probably snatch a piece of bread for herself on the way back. At midday she would rush back to feed the baby and then work on until 5.30pm. This went on day after day until mother and baby were completely debilitated.

Burnley is one of three Lancashire towns—Burnley, Nelson, and Colne—situated side by side on the western slope of the Pennine Hills (fig 10.2). The towns developed in the last century as centres for cotton weaving. Most of Burnley is in the valley where the rivers Brun and Calder meet. Nelson and Colne lie above it. For the six miles from the centre of Burnley through Nelson to Colne, there is hardly a break in the line of houses. For many years there have been large differences in the death rates in the towns.[1] In Burnley adult mortality rates are among the highest for any of the large towns in England and Wales, the standardised mortality ratio for all causes being 121 (table 10.1). In Colne the mortality rate is

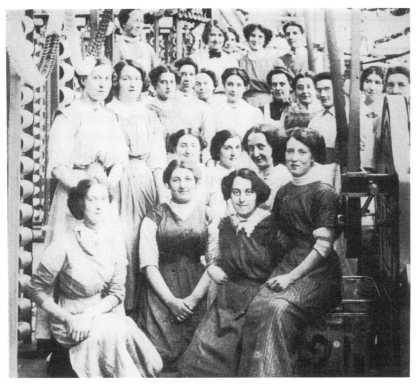

FIG 10.1—*Women weavers at Tulketh Mill about 1917.*

only 9% above the national average (standard mortality ratio, SMR = 109) whereas in Nelson, situated between the others, mortality is average (SMR = 100). Table 10.1 gives figures for a recent 11 year period. Eighty per cent of the excess mortality in Burnley is certified as being the result of coronary heart disease, chronic bronchitis, stroke, or bronchopneumonia. Mortality from cancer in the towns is around the national average, and mortality from lung cancer, an index of cigarette smoking, is average or below average.

The close proximity of the towns precludes explaining the large differences in mortality in terms of environmental influences such as rainfall. It is also unlikely that there are important differences in medical care; the hospital services for the towns are centred on Burnley. Instead the effect of socioeconomic factors is suggested. Recent census data show all three towns to be among the poorer towns in England and Wales, as indicated by the high percentage of manual workers, poor housing, and low income.[3] Socioeconomic differences between Nelson and Burnley are, however, small and less than the differences from the national average (table 10.2).

141

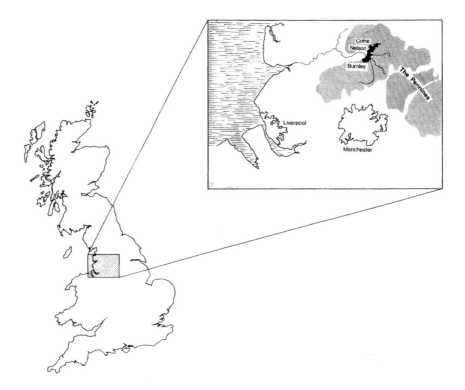

FIG 10.2—*Map of Great Britain showing the location of Burnley, Nelson, and Colne.*

It is of interest that Nelson has the greatest excess of manual workers but nevertheless has a death rate from all causes that is equal to the national average.

The present similarity of the towns belies the large differences that formerly existed and led to large differences in mortality among infants and young children. Table 10.3 shows infant mortality rates in the towns

TABLE 10.1—*Three Lancashire towns: standardised mortality ratios for causes of death at ages 55–74 years in 1968–78 (both sexes)*

Cause of death	Nelson	Colne	Burnley
All causes	100	109	121
Coronary heart disease	106	119	120
Chronic bronchitis	134	132	188
Pneumonia	108	125	174
Stroke	101	121	120
Lung cancer	81	83	100
Other cancers	90	106	101
Other causes	97	93	117

TABLE 10.2—*Three Lancashire towns: socioeconomic indices in 1971 compared with those in England and Wales*

	Nelson	Colne	Burnley	England and Wales
Employed men in social classes (%)				
I	2	3	3	5
II	13	14	13	18
III, non-manual	8	10	10	12
III, manual	48	47	45	38
IV	18	16	20	18
V	11	11	10	9
Households with exclusive use of all amenities (%)*	67	72	63	82
People living more than one person per room (%)	14	10	14	12
Households in dwellings of less than five rooms (%)	55	44	51	36
Households owning a car (%)	40	36	34	52
Infant mortality per 1000 1968–72	20	19	22	18
Total population	31 249	18 940	76 513	

*Hot water, fixed bath, inside lavatory.

for four periods from 1896 to 1925.[45] Throughout this time rates rose from Nelson to Colne to Burnley. Rates in Burnley were considerably above the average for England and Wales, and were consistently among the highest of any town. Data for 1911–13 distinguish neonatal and postneonatal deaths; rates rose between Nelson and Burnley for both

TABLE 10.3—*Three Lancashire towns: infant mortality rates per 1000 births from 1896 to 1925, child mortality and birth rate from 1911 to 1913*

	Nelson	Colne	Burnley	England and Wales
Infant mortality per 1000 births, 1896–1925:				
1896–98	154	170	197	155
1907–10	107	130	171	113
1911–13	87	130	177	111
1921–25	79	109	114	76
Rates from 1911 to 1913:				
Infant mortality per 1000 births:				
Neonatal	38	37	49	
Postneonatal	49	93	128	
Cause:				
Group of five diseases*	35	33	53	
Bronchitis and pneumonia	17	25	26	
Diarrhoea	16	30	48	
Mortality at age 1–5 years per 1000 survivors at age one year	58	85	96	
Birth rate per 1000 population	18	21	23	

*See text.

neonatal and postneonatal deaths, and for deaths from the three main groups of causes, that is, the so called "group of five" diseases, bronchitis and pneumonia, and diarrhoea. The "group of five" diseases were premature birth, congenital defects, birth injury, lack of breast milk, and marasmus: the most common of these were premature birth and congenital defects. Differences in mortality between the towns persisted through early childhood to five years of age. The birth rate also rose from Nelson to Colne to Burnley.

SOCIAL CONDITIONS IN THE PAST

We have an unusually detailed knowledge of social conditions in the towns at the beginning of the century because they were described in a report of the Local Government Board in 1914.[5] The generation whose infancy is described in this report belong to those whose death rates are shown in table 10.1. In all three towns the level of employment was high, and wages were relatively good. The staple industry was cotton weaving, and the textile industry employed 40% of all the women and girls aged 10 years and over. Many of the women who worked in the weaving mills of Burnley and Colne were from the second or third generation of Lancashire industrial workers. Nelson, however, had developed more recently and had an eightfold increase in population between 1871 and 1911. Most of the people were immigrants from adjacent areas, especially from rural parts of Yorkshire.

> This fact has an important bearing on the question of infantile mortality, owing to the general good health and the habits of cleanliness and thrift characteristic of these immigrants from rural districts.

The women were described as "sturdier and healthier" than those in Burnley.

There were no crêches at the mills. Usually the return of the mothers to work was soon followed by complete weaning and the infant, together with other children in the family below school age, was placed in the care of an untrained "minder" who was paid by the mother.

> In view of the fact that so many mothers are anxious, for the sake of the wages, to get back to employment in the mills as soon as possible after childbirth, a large proportion of children born in Burnley are deprived of the advantages of breast feeding after the first few weeks of life—... In Colne and still more in Nelson breast feeding is usually continued longer than in Burnley.

Most houses in the towns were built of stone. In Nelson, however, houses were newer and had more rooms (table 10.4), and so were less crowded. The worst houses were the back to back houses in the oldest parts of Burnley and Colne, which were small, had no means of ventilation to the outside air, and lacked facilities for the storage of food and milk. Infant

144

TABLE 10.4—*Three Lancashire towns: housing conditions, mean family size, and total population, 1911*

	Nelson	Colne	Burnley	England and Wales
Percentage of population in dwellings of less than four rooms	5·6	15·1	13·6	19·4
Percentage of population living more than two persons to a room	3·7	6·6	9·5	9·1
Percentage (no.) of dwellings back to back or single room	0·6 (52)	17·0 (1000)	9·9 (2371)	—
Mean family size	4·3	4·3	4·4	4·4
Total population	39 479	25 689	106 322	

mortality was much higher in such houses—248 per 1000 in the back to back houses of Colne during 1912, for example, compared with 80 in the so called "through" houses. Much of this excess mortality was the result of diarrhoea. Resettlement of families from back to back houses to "through" houses was accompanied by a fall in infant mortality to around the average for "through" houses, showing that high mortality was a consequence of the structure of the houses rather than of the habits of those who occupied them.

Sanitary conditions in Nelson were better than those in the other two towns. In Nelson the women kept the streets outside their houses clean, "more water being said to be used for this purpose in Nelson than in any other town in Lancashire". In Nelson communal pits, used for disposal of household refuse, were small and covered and were "in striking contrast" to the large open pits in Burnley and Colne, which favoured the breeding of flies. Refuse collected from the pits and bins in Nelson and Colne was destroyed, whereas in Burnley around half was put on to "tips", which were sites for breeding flies. In Nelson, and to a lesser extent Colne, the manure pits around stables and cowsheds were disinfected in summer to prevent flies breeding. Sanitary regulations for the production and sale of milk were more strictly enforced in Nelson.

SUMMARY

The past differences in infant mortality among the three towns can be linked to differences in the health and physique of mothers, infant feeding practices, housing, and sanitation. They were not related to differences in income or occupation. The children born to the "sturdier and healthier" mothers in Nelson, more of whom were breast fed, now have lower death rates from cardiovascular disease. After birth these children lived in better, less crowded houses and now have lower death rates from chronic bronchitis.

Mothers in Nelson had better health and physique because it was a newer town. The people were recent migrants from nearby rural areas rather than second or third generation industrial workers. The effects of life in towns in reducing the fitness of successive generations was described by Charles Booth[6] in his *Life and Labour of the People in London*, based on surveys carried out from 1886 onwards.

London[7]

For more than a hundred years, people living in the cities and large towns of Britain have had higher death rates than people living in small towns and villages.[8] London is an exception. During 1980–85, for example, standardised mortality ratios for all causes in London, expressed in relation to a national average of 100, were 96 among men and 93 among women. These low standardised mortality ratios resulted largely from low rates of cardiovascular disease. Ratios for coronary heart disease were 90 in men and 87 in women; ratios for stroke were 78 in each sex. Londoners' low cardiovascular death rates have never been explained.

The geographical distribution of national death rates during 1968–78 has been analysed in unusual detail.[9] During this period, standardised mortality ratios in London for coronary heart disease and stroke combined were 87 in men and 83 in women. In none of the 33 London boroughs was cardiovascular mortality above the national average in either sex. London's low cardiovascular mortality contrasts with above average mortality from diseases associated with poor socioeconomic conditions, cigarette smoking, and alcohol consumption. Standardised mortality ratios during 1968–78 were: for chronic bronchitis 105 in men and 111 in women; for lung cancer, 114 and 127; for cirrhosis of the liver, 101 and 103; and for suicide, 115 and 130. In only four of the 33 boroughs were lung cancer death rates below the national average, the lowest standardised mortality ratio being 92. Thus the lifestyle of Londoners does not seem especially healthy and is not consistent with their low death rates from cardiovascular disease.

In the early years of this century London had low rates of maternal and neonatal mortality. Maternal mortality during 1911–14, for example, was 3·1 per 1000 births compared with 4·0 in England and Wales. Neonatal mortality was 33 per 1000 births compared with 39. In the past, maternal mortality was low in places where women had good physique, nutrition, and health, and neonatal mortality was low where few babies had low birthweight.[10 11] The low maternal and neonatal mortality in London therefore implies that, at the beginning of this century, its women had good physique, health, and nutrition, which is surprising. It conflicts with the picture of London presented by novelists, and with detailed descriptions of life in London given by the surveys which Charles Booth carried out from 1886 onwards. Writing of the London poor, he said,[6] "Their life is the life of savages with vicissitudes of extreme hardship and occasional

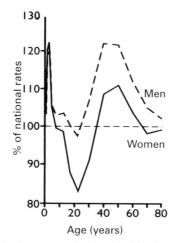

FIG 10.3—*Age specific death rates in London, 1901–10, expressed as a percentage of national rates for England and Wales.*

excess. Their food is of the coarsest description, and their only luxury is drink". Amid this savagery, pregnancy, childbirth, and early infancy were unusually safe for both the mother and the baby. Why?

SOCIAL CONDITIONS IN THE PAST

Young women in London had remarkably low death rates at the beginning of the century. These low rates contrasted with the high rates in girls under 15. Fig 10.3 shows age specific death rates among women in London during 1901–10, expressed as a percentage of the rates in England and Wales. [7] Among girls under five years of age London rates were above the national average, and 20% above in girls aged 2–3 years. With increasing age the rates for girls and women fell sharply so that from 15 to 34 years they were well below the average, and 17% below in girls aged 20–24. Among older women rates rose and were again above the average. Among men the overall pattern was similar to that in women, with lower rates in young adults; however, only at ages 15–24 were London rates below the national average. Analysis of death rates for the previous decade, 1891–1900, shows a similar pattern.[12]

Fig 10.4 compares death rates in girls under 15 years of age in the counties of England and Wales with death rates in young women aged 15–34 years. As expected the rates are related. Counties with lower death rates in girls, which are mostly in the south and east of the country, have lower rates in young women, and vice versa. London is exceptional. The high death rate in girls is disproportionate to the low rate in young women.

The main causes of death of young women in London, and the relation of London death rates to national rates, are shown in table 10.5. London

147

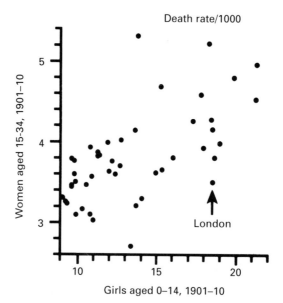

FIG 10.4—*Death rates among girls under 15 years and women aged 15–34 years in the counties of England and Wales 1901–10.*

women had low death rates from tuberculosis and other infectious diseases, and low mortality during childbirth. Analysis of death rates during the previous decade, 1891–1900, shows a similar pattern, with low death rates for tuberculosis and the major infectious diseases, and from childbirth, and high rates for cancer and violent death.[13]

At this time the death rates of London children from common infections, including measles and whooping cough, were the highest of any county in

TABLE 10.5—*Leading causes of death among women aged 15–34 years in London, 1901–10*

Cause of death	Death rate per million		London rates as percentage of England and Wales
	London	England and Wales	
Tuberculosis	1231	1485	83
Childbirth	288	386	75
Pneumonia	202	236	85
Cancer	131	97	134
Violence	130	120	108
Enteric fever	71	98	72
Septic diseases	69	40	174
Rheumatic fever	57	65	87
All other causes	1300	1381	94

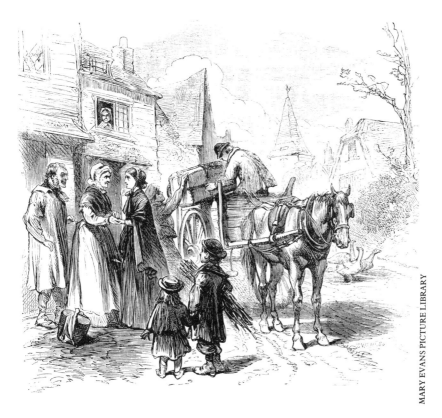

FIG 10.5—*Girls leaving the country to go into service were among the "the cream of the youth of the villages, travelling ... definitely to seek a known economic advantage". They made up over a fifth of the young women in London at the 1911 census.*

England and Wales. Booth described London children in the poorer classes as "underfed, ill-clad, badly lodged, and poorly born".[14] They lived where "the main streets, narrow at best, branch off into others narrower still; and these again into a labyrinth of blind alleys, courts and lanes; all dirty, foul-smelling, and littered with garbage of every kind. The houses are old, damp and dilapidated".[13]

Two possible explanations for the good health of young women in London are migration and domestic service.[7] Dwindling rural industries, the depression of agriculture, and low wages in the villages encouraged young people to migrate to the towns. Those in the southern counties went in large numbers to London, attracted by the opportunities for employment and the high wages. The usual age of migration was between 15 and 30 years, and more young women than young men went to London, largely

MARY EVANS PICTURE LIBRARY

149

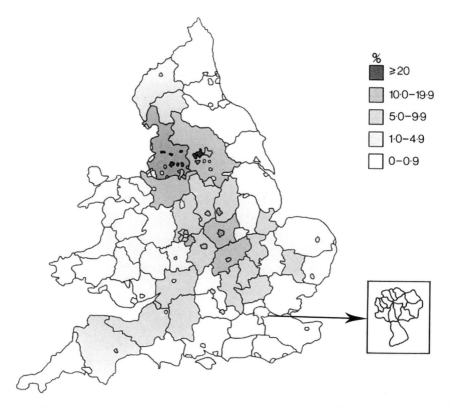

FIG 10.6—*Percentage of girls aged 10–14 years working in 1901 (not as domestic servants): administrative counties and county boroughs of England and Wales.*

because of the demand for domestic servants. This was reflected in the relative excess of young women in London's population which persisted through the eighteenth and nineteenth centuries.[15]

Booth described migration into London (fig 10.5):[13]

> The countrymen drawn in (to London) are mainly the cream of the youth of the villages, travelling not so often vaguely in search of work as definitely to seek a known economic advantage. . . . It is the result of the conditions of life in great towns, and especially in this the greatest town of all, that muscular strength and energy get gradually used up; the second generation of Londoners is of lower physique and has less power of persistent work than the first; and the third generation (where it exists) is lower than the second. . . . London is to a great extent nourished by the literal consumption of bone and sinew from the country; by the absorption every year of large numbers of persons of stronger physique, who leaven the whole mass, largely direct the industries, raise the standard of health and comfort, and keep up the rate of growth of the great city only to give place in their turn to a fresh set of recruits, after London life for one or two generations has reduced them to the level of those among whom they live.

Fig 10.6 shows that, although many girls in the north of England, especially Lancashire, were employed in industry from a young age, girls in London escaped this. Their usual employment was in domestic service. Thirty per cent of young women in employment in London were in domestic service at the time of the 1911 census. Women generally left domestic service when they married, and an unknown percentage of the young women who were married would have previously been in domestic service. Young women who went into domestic service would have had good nutrition in the years before their marriage and pregnancies.[16] The food given to domestic servants "was usually very good, and in all but very rare cases greatly superior to that obtainable by the other members of the working class families from which servants are drawn".[17] When members of the Domestic Servants Society, formed in 1912, applied for health insurance, they were found to be more healthy than any other group of women workers.[18]

During routine examinations of London schoolchildren around the time of the First World War the girls were more likely than boys to be classed as having "excellent nutrition".[19] This contrasted with findings in industrial towns, where boys were fed better than girls. In Hull, for example, during 1913 "the proportion of boys classed as enjoying 'good' nutrition far exceeded the proportion of girls so classed ... by a factor of five among the 10 year old children".[20] Girls in London seemed to escape the unequal division of the family's food which occurred in industrial Britain because of the emphasis on male manual work. Unequal division of food in favour of the man still occurs elsewhere in the world, in patrilineal societies, and in societies where veneration of ancestors is centred on men.

SUMMARY

The health of young women in London at the beginning of the century was unusually good because many were born in the fertile agricultural counties of southern England or had mothers who were born in these counties. They therefore had good nutrition in fetal life and infancy. Among children in London there was no preferential feeding of boys. Girls who went into domestic service were unusually well fed in adolescence and as young adults. The children born to these young women today have low death rates from cardiovascular disease. After birth these children lived in poor, overcrowded houses and today have high death rates from chronic bronchitis.

Lessons from history

The studies of socioeconomic conditions in three Lancashire towns and London add little to the evidence that the prenatal and early postnatal environment have a major effect on cardiovascular disease and other disorders. This evidence rests on follow up studies of thousands of people, described in this book. Lancashire and London do, however, give an insight into past social changes which may have determined patterns of mortality today. They allow conclusions which go beyond such general statements as that of the Black Report on inequalities of health in Britain:[21] "Much, we feel, can only be understood in terms of the more diffuse consequences of the class structure."

Migration from the countryside into the expanding industrial towns in Britain was associated with a worsening of the diet:[22] "Take indifferently twenty well-fed husbandmen, and compare them with twenty industrial workers who have equal means of support" Thackrah wrote in 1832 "and the superiority of the agricultural peasants in health, vigour and size will be obvious". We do not know in any detail how the diet in industrial towns at the turn of the century was deficient. There is, however, anecdotal evidence.

In a recent survey of elderly women in six areas of England, a woman who worked in Hertfordshire as an upstairs maid in the 1920s described her diet:[16]

> We had four wonderful meals a day and it was comfort from the word go ... An excellent breakfast of porridge, egg dishes or bacon. Lunch was always meat and vegetables and a pudding of sorts. Tea was bread and butter and cake, and supper was usually cold meat, bubble and squeak or a cheese dish. I must say when I got married I thought, "Oh dear, I don't like this poverty," after living in so much comfort.

The daughter of a labourer growing up in Sheffield at the same time recalled:

> I didn't go hungry but we'd no luxuries. Breakfast and tea would be bread and butter mostly. On a Sunday morning we had a bit of cooked bacon, when my dad was working, just a little bit like that and my dad's words were, "Now then, little bits of bacon and big lumps of bread."

The general picture given by studies such as this is of girls and young women in industrial areas eating fewer meals a day, and having less red meat, fruit, and vegetables. If their mothers had grown up in an industrial area the girls would have been undernourished *in utero*. This would further impair their ability to sustain fetal growth in their own offspring (page 122). In areas where there was little employment for women, notably many coal mining areas, girls married young and had large families, which may have further compounded fetal undernutrition.

Summary

History suggests that today's inequalities in health are linked to poor maternal and infant health in the past. It endorses the findings from follow up studies of men and women, and experiments on animals, described in this book. To prevent disease in the next generation we need to direct our attention to the nutrition of mothers and their babies and to exposure to infection in early childhood.

1 Barker DJP, Osmond C. Inequalities in health in Britain: specific explanations in three Lancashire towns. *BMJ* 1987; **294**:749–52.

2 Harris Museum and Art Gallery. *The story of Preston.* Preston, 1992.

3 Census Office. *Census of England and Wales 1901.* London: HMSO, 1917.

4 Local Government Board. *Forty second annual report, 1912–13.* Supplement in continuation of the report of the medical officer of the board for 1912–13. London: HMSO, 1913.

5 Local Government Board. *Forty third annual report, 1913–14.* Supplement in continuation of the report of the medical officer of the board for 1913–14. London: HMSO, 1914.

6 Booth C. *Life and labour of the people in London.* First series: *Poverty.* Volume 1, *East, central and south London.* London: Macmillan, 1902.

7 Barker DJP, Osmond C, Pannett B. Why Londoners have low death rates from ischaemic heart disease and stroke. *BMJ* 1992;**305**:1551–4.

8 *Registrar General's statistical review of England and Wales.* Part 1: tables, medical. London: HMSO, 1880 and following years.

9 Gardner MJ, Winter PD, Barker DJP. Atlas of mortality from selected diseases in England and Wales 1968–78. Chichester: Wiley, 1984.

10 Campbell JM, Cameron D, Jones DM. High maternal mortality in certain areas. London: HMSO, 1932. (Ministry of Health reports on public health and medical subjects No 68.)

11 Local Government Board. Thirty-ninth annual report 1909–10. Supplement to the report of the board's medical officer. Supplement on infant and child mortality. London: HMSO, 1910.

12 *Registrar General of Births, Deaths and Marriages in England and Wales.* Supplement to the sixty fifth annual report. Part 1, Registration summary tables 1891–1900. London: HMSO, 1907.

13 Booth C. *Life and labour of the people in London.* Second series: *Industry in London* volume 5. *Comparisons, survey and conclusions.* London: Macmillan, 1903.

14 Booth C. *Life and Labour of the people in London.* First series: *Poverty in London.* Volume 3. *Blocks of buildings, schools and immigration.* London: Macmillan, 1902.

15 Earle P. *A City Full of People. Men and Women of London 1650–1750.* London: Methuen, 1994.

16 Fellague Ariouat J, Barker DJP. The diet of girls and young women at the beginning of the century. *Nutrition and Health* 1993;**9**:15–23.

17 Booth C. *Life and labour of the people in London.* Second series: *Industry in London.* Volume 4. *Public professional and domestic service, unsuccessful classes.* London: Macmillan, 1903.

18 *The new survey of London life and labour.* Volume II. *London industries.* London: PS King and Son, 1931.

19 London County Council. *Annual report of council 1915–19.* Volume III, *Public health.* London: LCC, 1919.

20 Wall R. *Some inequalities in the raising of boys and girls in nineteenth and twentieth-century England and Wales*. Cambridge: Cambridge Group for the History of Population and Social Structure, 1990.
21 Townsend P, Davidson N. *Inequalities of health: the Black report*. Harmondsworth: Penguin, 1982.
22 Thackrah CT. *The effects of arts, trades and professions and of civic states and the habits of living on health and longevity with suggestions for the removal of many of the agents which produce disease and shorten the duration of life*, London: Longman, 1832.

11: Preventing disease: the future

A hundred years ago, when most people lived in the countryside, the importance of good nourishment for the long term wellbeing of the young was widely recognised. In 1830, when Mary McCraicen, secretary of the ladies committee of the Belfast Poorhouse, was appealing for money she wrote "Health and consequent comfort and well-being through life depends in a great measure on proper nourishment and treatment during the period of infancy". The adverse effects of industrialisation on fetal growth did not go unremarked at the time. The *Encyclopaedia Britannica* for 1884 states:

> The building up of the placenta by the mother and the performance of the function of that wonderful organ require certain favouring conditions. These are certainly not to be found in factory labour.

Death rates in generations

In the past when tuberculosis and rheumatic fever were common, the proposition that health in childhood determined health in adult life was self evident. In the 1920s records of annual death rates in Britain had accumulated over sufficient years to allow the link between childhood and adult disease rates to be examined statistically.[1] It was found that over the previous 80 years death rates at different ages had begun to fall at different times. Rates in the young began to fall earlier than those in the old. Derrick[2] showed that if death rates at each age were plotted by year of birth, that is, by generation, there was a remarkably regular pattern. Each succeeding generation displayed a lower mortality at all ages from childhood to old age. He concluded that "each generation is endowed with a vitality peculiarly its own, which persistently manifests itself through the succeeding stages of its existence".[2]

In the years up to the Second World War the existence of strong generation or "cohort" effects on mortality was examined and confirmed.[3] Discussions of what caused them sought to apportion responsibility between genetic influences and the environment during childhood and adolescence. Seemingly uninformed by much knowledge of biology this statistical debate, which has been reviewed by Kuh and Davey Smith,[1] led to no conclusions. It did, however, establish the importance of generation effects in public health policy. Watt and Ecob[4] have recently re-emphasised this by comparing death rates in the two major cities in Scotland: Edinburgh, the capital, and the less affluent Glasgow. They found that in successive generations death rates in Glasgow were higher at all adult ages, and people in Glasgow experienced the same mortality rates as people in Edinburgh 3·6 years earlier in men and 3·9 years earlier in women:[5 6]

> For the same chronological age, Glaswegians are about four years older than people in Edinburgh. At any given age Glaswegians have more miles on the clock.

The existence of generation effects is important in relating the time trends of specific diseases to past trends in maternal and infant nutrition.

Trends in diseases

From the middle of the last century, in Britain and elsewhere, a succession of public health reforms began to improve conditions for mothers and their babies.[7] Increased intakes of total calories, animal fat, fruit and fresh vegetables, vitamins, and minerals led to better early growth. Improvements in sanitation and housing, and reduction in family size and overcrowding, led mortality from infectious diseases to fall. Infant mortality began to decline at the turn of the century (fig 11.1), and fell almost without interruption from 152 per 1000 births in 1900 to 8 per 1000 live births in 1990. Neonatal and postneonatal death rates both fell, but the environment during infancy improved more rapidly than the intrauterine environment, and the proportion of deaths occurring in the neonatal period doubled.

To establish whether the improvements in fetal and infant nutrition and health that were reflected in the fall in infant mortality are now apparent in falling rates of adult disease, it is useful to divide adult diseases into three groups. These may be called diseases of poverty, diseases of affluence, and diseases of change.[8]

DISEASES OF POVERTY

The incidences of diseases associated with poor living standards, which include tuberculosis and rheumatic fever, have declined during this century. Stroke and chronic bronchitis can be included with this group for they too are most common in the least affluent areas and in people with the lowest incomes, and their incidence has fallen during the last 50 years.[9-12]

Death from *stroke* occurs at an older age than death from coronary heart disease, and there are as yet insufficient deaths in the longitudinal studies in Hertfordshire and Sheffield to allow definite conclusions about the association between stroke and early growth. Death rates show trends with birthweight similar to those of coronary heart disease, but they are not statistically significant (unpublished). Findings from geography and studies

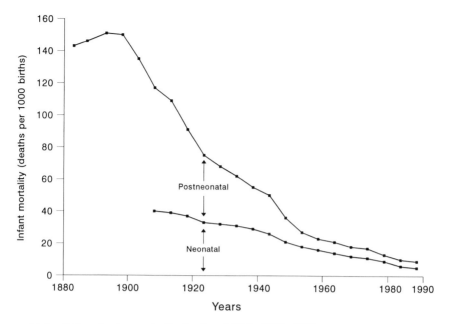

FIG 11.1—*Infant death rates in England and Wales 1883–1990.*

of risk factors for stroke, however, point to its origin *in utero*. Death rates from stroke correlate geographically with past maternal and neonatal mortality, though not with postneonatal mortality (see chapter 1). High blood pressure and plasma fibrinogen concentrations, the two major known antecedents of stroke, are both strongly related to impaired growth *in utero* (see chapters 4 and 5).

From this it follows that improvements in the intrauterine environment, which led in Britain to a fall in neonatal mortality, should be reflected in a later decline in death rates from stroke. Fig 11.2 shows the age specific mortality from stroke for the period 1950–84.[12] Death rates declined continuously so that, by the end of the period, rates among men had halved and among women had fallen to three eighths of their 1950 levels. These data are consistent with generation effects, each successive generation having lower rates at each age than the one before. The fall in death rates from stroke began before the widespread use of anti-hypertensive therapy but may now be hastened by it.

Chronic bronchitis is linked to impaired lung growth *in utero* and during infancy and to infections of the lower respiratory tract during early childhood (chapter 7). It follows that past improvements in maternal nutrition and health, improvements in housing, and reduction in family size and over-

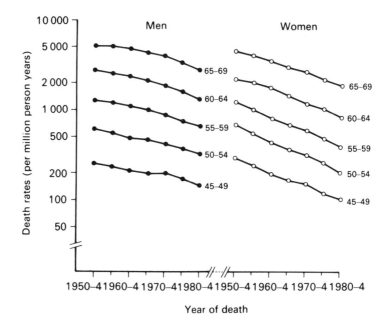

FIG 11.2—*Age specific mortality from stroke, England and Wales, 1950–84 (ICD 8th revision, Codes 431–438).*

crowding should be reflected in a later decline in chronic bronchitis. In Britain age specific mortality from chronic bronchitis has fallen progressively over the last 50 years.[9] Osmond[10] has shown that the trends are made up of two components: a "cohort" value, summarising the mortality experience of a generation, and a "period" value summarising the experience of all age groups at one point in time. Figs 11.3 and 11.4 show these two components in men and women.[11]

The "cohort" component rises and falls and corresponds remarkably closely to that found for lung cancer. It may be attributed to the smoking habits of successive generations. These differed in men and women. The "period" component, defined by year of death, declines steeply, age specific death rates falling progressively from 1941. This pattern is quite different to that found for lung cancer, for which the period values were almost constant. It is consistent with chronic bronchitis being linked to early growth and infection whereas lung cancer is not (see table 7.1). The steeper fall among women than men is consistent with the smaller contribution of smoking to their mortality. Improved treatment after the advent of antibiotics may have contributed to the decline in both sexes.

The Clean Air Act 1956 was not followed by a change in the rate of decline of chronic bronchitis. This suggests that chronic air pollution in adult life, as opposed to short episodes of high pollution, may be a less

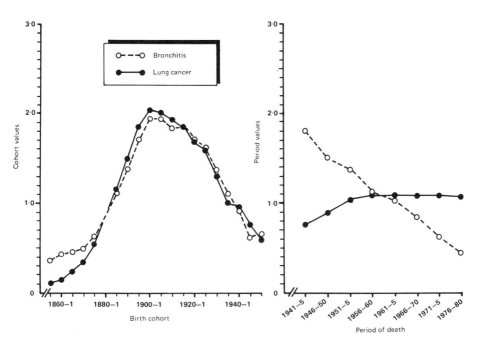

FIG 11.3—*Cohort and period of death values for chronic bronchitis and lung cancer in men aged over 25 in England and Wales during 1941–80.*

important cause of mortality from bronchitis than previously supposed. A survey of respiratory symptoms in a sample of British adults showed that, in the absence of cigarette smoking, the influence of air pollution was small.[13] There is suggestive evidence that children exposed to high levels of air pollution may have an increased risk of serious respiratory disease, but this is not conclusive. One inconsistency is the high rates for respiratory disease recorded in South Wales at a time when air pollution was relatively low.[14 15]

DISEASES OF AFFLUENCE

The second group of diseases is associated with affluence. Such diseases are more common among more prosperous people living in more prosperous areas, and their incidence is rising. They include obesity, gallstones, renal stones, and cancers of the breast, ovary, and prostate.[8 9] Little is known about how fetal and infant development influences these diseases, though there is suggestive evidence, including findings in the Dutch Hunger Winter that link fetal undernutrition to adult obesity (page 22). A recent hypothesis proposed that breast cancer begins *in utero*.[16] Although a comparison of the birth records of women with breast cancer and controls in Sweden

159

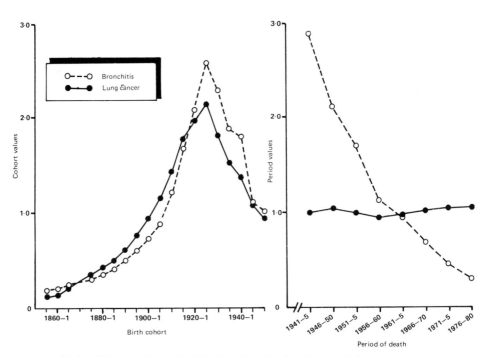

FIG 11.4—*Cohort and period of death values for chronic bronchitis and lung cancer in women aged over 25 in England and Wales during 1941–80.*

showed that the risk of the disease increased with increasing birthweight and birth length, the findings were not statistically significant.[17] Further support for the hypothesis comes, however, from a geographical study in England and Wales where counties with taller populations have lower mortality from cardiovascular disease but higher mortality from three hormone related cancers: of the breast, prostate, and ovary.[18] These findings could suggest that promotion of early growth has disadvantages as well as benefits.

DISEASES OF CHANGE

The third group of diseases is at different times associated with poverty and affluence. It includes coronary heart disease, acute appendicitis, and duodenal ulcer. In the early part of this century these diseases were more common among the rich and their incidence rose. Later, they became more common among the poor and their incidence fell.

The term *Western diseases* is used to describe a group of diseases that are common in industrialised countries, but uncommon elsewhere, whose incidence rises with the start of industrialisation.[19] As these diseases appear to be a consequence of industrialisation, it is argued that their prevention

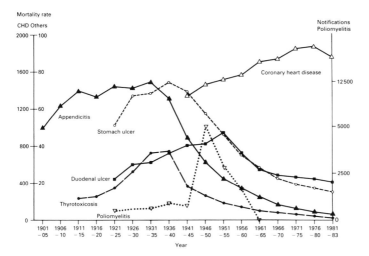

FIG 11.5—*Average annual mortality rate from selected diseases in England and Wales from 1901, and numbers of notifications of poliomyelitis in five year periods.*

must depend on a return to practices of the past—for example, resumption of a diet high in complex carbohydrates and low in animal fats. Yet "Western" diseases include both diseases of affluence and diseases of change, whose incidence has fallen whilst the environmental changes of industrialisation have persisted. Thyrotoxicosis serves as a model to examine how the incidence of a disease may rise and fall without a matching increase and decrease in exposure to any environmental influence.

Figure 11.5 shows death rates in England and Wales from a number of diseases of change, and includes death rates from thyrotoxicosis, which rose to a peak in the 1930s and thereafter declined. Most deaths from thyrotoxicosis occur in the elderly, among whom toxic multinodular goitre is the usual cause. Analyses of age specific rates in successive generations show that they rose progressively in people born after 1836, and reached a peak in those born between 1871 and 1886.[20] This is shown in fig 11.6, which gives rates in each generation according to their year of birth.

Figure 11.6 also shows the progressive increase in dietary iodine in Britain during this century, as a consequence of diversification of diet and availability of iodine in many foods including fish, meat, and milk.[21] Iodine deficiency during childhood was widespread among people born in Britain in the 1800s. Successive generations, however, were exposed to more iodine in adult life. There is evidence that people who are iodine deficient in youth are less able to adapt to increased iodine intake in later life and tend

161

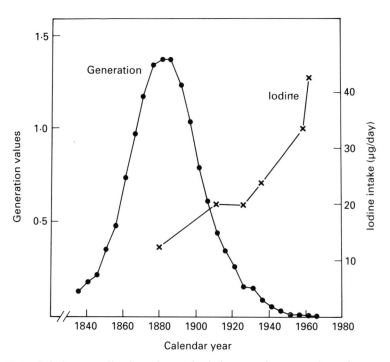

FIG 11.6—*Relative mortality from thyrotoxicosis in successive generations of women in England and Wales, according to year of birth, and estimated per capita daily iodine intake from milk, meat, and fish.*

to develop thyrotoxicosis.[22] This would explain the rise in deaths from thyrotoxicosis in the early part of this century (fig 11.5). Successive generations born after 1880 were exposed to more iodine in childhood, which would have lessened their susceptibility to iodine in adult life; accordingly, thyrotoxicosis mortality fell from around 1940. This explanation of the time trends accounts for the apparent paradox that toxic nodular goitre is now common only in those areas of Britain where iodine deficiency used to be prevalent. The essential process thought to underlie the trends of occurrence of toxic nodular goitre is a response to an environmental influence during early life which has a critical effect on the ability to adapt to subsequent exposure. The same process could determine trends in coronary heart disease.

Coronary heart disease—Death from coronary heart disease was not distinguished from death from other forms of heart disease before 1940, but other evidence shows that rates rose steeply during the first part of the century. From 1940 death rates continued to rise and reached a plateau in the 1970s (fig 11.5). Since 1980 there has been a small decline. Similar

162

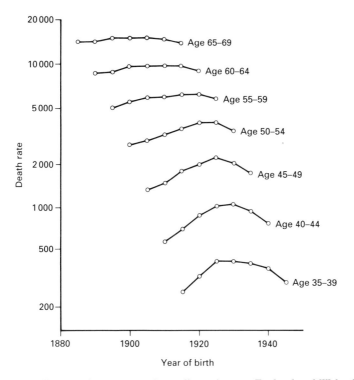

FIG 11.7—*Mortality rates from coronary heart disease in men, England and Wales during 1950–84.*

patterns occurred in the USA, Canada, Australia, and New Zealand; following steep increases there have been substantial falls—around one quarter in the last 20 years in the USA.[23] Although during this increase coronary heart disease was more common in wealthier people, it is now more common among people with lower incomes living in less affluent areas. The time trends of the disease may therefore depend on two groups of environmental causes: the first acting *in utero* and infancy and associated with poor living standards; and the second associated with affluence and perhaps mediated through a high energy, high fat diet. The rise in the disease results from an increase in the second; its fall from reduction in the first.

Figures 11.7 and 11.8 show age specific mortality from coronary heart disease, for the years 1950–84, plotted against year of birth. Among men, the generation born around 1925 had the highest death rates at all ages so far attained. Among women the picture is similar, although the peak is less clearly defined at 1925. The occurrence of a worst affected generation is

163

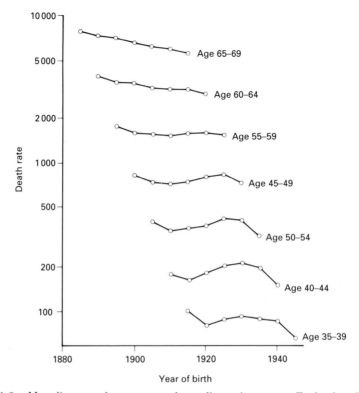

FIG 11.8—*Mortality rates from coronary heart disease in women, England and Wales during 1950–84.*

consistent with the hypothesis that coronary disease is determined by two sets of influences.

Although this hypothesis synthesises our new understanding of the role of fetal growth in coronary heart disease with more established ideas on the role of adult lifestyle, it is not necessary to invoke two sets of influences to explain the rise and fall of coronary heart disease or its changing rates in successive generations. Coronary heart disease does not seem to be associated with proportionate or symmetrical growth retardation, resulting from undernutrition in early gestation, but is associated with disproportionate growth retardation, which results from undernutrition in mid or late gestation and leads to either thinness at birth or a short body in relation to head size. This is consistent with the different patterns of fetal growth that occur in different countries. An important difference between fetal growth in the less developed and that in Western countries is that symmetrical growth retardation is common in less developed countries, whereas asymmetrical growth retardation prevails in Western countries.[24]

TABLE 11.1—*Mean birthweight, head circumference, length, and ponderal index of babies born at term in different countries*

Country	Place	No. of babies	Birthweight (kg)	Head circumference (cm)	Length (cm)	Ponderal index (kg/cm³)
China	Chendu	543	3·33	33·5	49·1	28·1
India	New Delhi	550	2·97	34·2	49·7	24·2
Sweden	Uppsala	597	3·74	35·8	51·7	27·1

Table 11.1 shows the birth measurements of newborn babies who were included in the WHO study of lactational amenorrhoea (unpublished data). The babies in China have smaller heads and are shorter but fatter, as indicated by ponderal index, than babies in India or Sweden. The Chinese babies are symmetrically small babies (see fig 9.2). The babies in New Delhi are, however, thin, as has been observed elsewhere in India.[25]

One can infer that in China mothers are chronically undernourished, and babies become undernourished early in gestation and reduce their growth rates. They are thereby protected from undernutrition in later gestation (page 19) and are born fat. They are not prone to coronary heart disease as adults but have high death rates from stroke.[26] In India mothers are less severely undernourished and the fetus does not become undernourished until mid-gestation. It has a larger head and is longer but undernutrition makes it thin at birth with less skeletal muscle. It is prone to non-insulin dependent diabetes. In Western communities mothers are better nourished but fetal undernutrition in late gestation leads to preservation of brain growth at the expense of the trunk, including the liver. Adults have disordered lipid metabolism and blood clotting, which are regulated by the liver, and are prone to coronary heart disease.

Under this hypothesis coronary heart disease represents a stage of improving nutrition between chronic maternal malnutrition and nutrition at a plane that allows the mother to nourish her fetus adequately throughout gestation. This offers an economical though speculative interpretation of the time trends of coronary heart disease. It suggests that, except in so far as it affects maternal nutrition, adult lifestyle is not closely linked to the time trends of the disease, although it contributes to the rates of disease within a population.

Non-insulin dependent diabetes—This is not strictly a "Western" disease because it is common in some developing countries including India.[27] Its incidence, however, rises steeply with industrialisation, and the highest known prevalences are in populations which have become "Westernised" unusually rapidly (page 90). It is uncertain whether the prevalence has changed recently in the Western World.[28] The disease is associated with undernutrition *in utero* and obesity in adult life (chapter 6). One could therefore predict that its incidence will rise and fall as nutrition in a population improves. The initial rise will result from an increase in adult obesity, and the fall will occur when reduced fetal undernutrition becomes reflected in better glucose/insulin metabolism in adult life. Table 6.3 showed how better growth *in utero* and during infancy protected against the effects of obesity on plasma glucose concentrations.

Findings which support this model come from a recent survey of the Nauruan Islanders; following its steep post-war rise the prevalence of non-insulin dependent diabetes is now falling.[29] The fall has occurred in people born after 1945, and has not been accompanied by any change in the prevalence of obesity or other risk factors for diabetes related to adult lifestyle.

Poliomyelitis—Figure 11.5 shows the trend in notification rates for poliomyelitis in England and Wales. The disease was rare before this century but, as in other countries, it began to appear as hygienic and general living standards improved. This contrasts with the other common infectious diseases, which declined at this time. There was a sharp rise in notifications of poliomyelitis after the Second World War which persisted until the introduction of large scale immunisation. It is now known that the rise of poliomyelitis resulted from the increasing vulnerability of the central nervous system to poliovirus infection with increasing age. As hygiene, sanitation, and housing improved, the proportion of children escaping infection during the relatively safe period of infancy rose, and the number of cases of paralytic disease at later ages therefore rose in parallel.

Acute appendicitis—The outbreaks of appendicitis which have accompanied industrialisation in many parts of the world can similarly be explained as an age dependent consequence of infection. The so called "hygiene hypothesis" for acute appendicitis was described in chapter 8. In England and Wales, death rates from appendicitis increased abruptly and steeply from around 1900, and then fell progressively from the 1930s onwards (see fig 11.5). There is strong evidence that this trend reflected similar changes in incidence of the disease, and the same trends were recorded in other European countries and in the USA. The explanation of these trends is thought to lie in the reduced levels of enteric infection in young children brought about by better hygiene, making them liable to develop appendicitis in response to infections at a later age. With continued improvements in hygiene, exposure to infection throughout childhood and early adult life became less common. Because the appendix seems to be less vulnerable to infection after about 30 years of age, appendicitis declined.

Duodenal ulcer—Death rates from duodenal ulcer rose and fell in a similar way to those from acute appendicitis (see fig 11.5). The distribution of duodenal ulcer with social class was similar to appendicitis; while it was increasing it was more common among the rich, but as it declined it became more common in poorer people. Recent findings of organisms similar to *Campylobacter* sp. in peptic ulcers suggest that the disease is spread by an infective agent.[30] The time trends point to age dependent consequences of this infection.

Optimal rates of environmental change

Coronary heart disease, non-insulin dependent diabetes, appendicitis, and duodenal ulcer seem to rise and fall in response to the environmental changes that accompany industrialisation. These diseases characterise the change from a rural to an industrial society, and there is increasing evidence that they originate in responses to the early environment, including adaptation to nutrition during fetal life and age dependent consequences of infection. Hitherto the search for causes of "Western" diseases has concentrated on the adult environment. The importance of the fetal and infant environment in determining responses throughout life has been underestimated. Models of disease based on the effects of cigarette smoking, an influence in the adult environment which has been intensively studied, may have limited general application. Where differences in individuals' susceptibility to disease cannot be explained by differences in the adult environment, as is the case for coronary heart disease, they have often been attributed to genetic causes—especially if the disease has a familial tendency. Part of what was regarded as the genetic contribution to coronary heart disease and other disorders can now be attributed to the intrauterine or early postnatal environment.

Critical adaptations during early life may determine optimal rates of environmental change within populations. Appendicitis and duodenal ulcer became common at an early stage of improvements in hygiene. The size of epidemics of these diseases may depend on the speed with which hygiene improves throughout the population. The rise of appendicitis in Britain can be linked to the introduction of domestic hot water systems. The introduction of piped water supplies was spread over more than half a century, piped water not reaching some rural areas until after the Second World War. Swifter execution of sanitary health reforms started in the nineteenth century might have reduced the incidence of this disease.

By contrast, critical adaptations to nutrition in early life which determine adult responses to nutrition, as occur in toxic nodular goitre and as are suspected in non-insulin dependent diabetes, may limit the extent of dietary change to which a generation can be exposed without adverse effects. Generations undernourished in early life are susceptible to these diseases if better nourished in later life. It is not known how important adult "overnutrition" is in determining coronary heart disease compared with fetal undernutrition (page 163). Nevertheless it seems clear that, during early industrialisation, improvements in living standards should be directed at mothers and their babies. Although the industrial revolution in Britain brought high wages to adults, children continued to grow up under-nourished, in large families, and in poor, overcrowded homes.

Steep increases in the incidence of "Western" diseases regularly follow industrialisation and the associated changes in diet and hygiene. Large scale migration into cities in the less developed countries has changed people's diet, but poor hygiene persists. Elsewhere, as in China, im-provements in hygiene have occurred with little change in the traditional diet. If more was known about the processes by which the environment in early life influences adult health, the nutritional and hygienic benefits which accompany industrial development might be maximised, and the rise in incidence of "Western" disease minimised.

Mothers and babies today

The epidemiological evidence which links fetal nutrition and hygiene in early life with adult disease necessarily depends on studies of people born many years ago. It can be argued, therefore, that inequalities in adult disease in the Western World, between rich and poor, between people living in one place and those in another, are a legacy of the past. Improvements in nutrition and hygiene during this century may have already determined falling disease rates in future generations and a lessening of inequalities. There is, however, considerable evidence against this comfortable point of view.

Table 6.7 showed the blood pressures of an unselected group of four-year-old children born in Salisbury, a prosperous town in southern England, during 1984–85. Irrespective of their current size, and of other influences such as their mothers' blood presure or smoking habits, those who were thin at birth had raised systolic pressure. By the time they were seven years old their ability to store and metabolise glucose was reduced. Seemingly a predisposition to develop hypertension and non-insulin diabetes is already apparent.

Law and colleagues[31] compared the size at birth of an unselected sample of more than a thousand babies born in Salisbury during 1991 with that of a similar sample born in Burnley, one of the less affluent industrial towns in northern England. Burnley has had high perinatal mortality (stillbirth and early neonatal deaths) since the beginning of the century. Burnley babies today are thinner, as measured by ponderal index and arm and abdominal circumferences, and have smaller head circumferences (table 11.2). Their placental weight : birthweight ratio is higher. The thinness of

TABLE 11.2—*Average size of babies born in two English towns, 1991*

	Burnley $(n=1544)$	Salisbury $(n=1025)$	Difference Burnley–Salisbury (95% confidence interval)
Birthweight	3342	3458	−166 (−154 to −77)
Crown–heel length (cm)	50·0	50·1	−0·1 (−0·3 to 0·04)
Ponderal index (kg/m³)	26·6	27·4	−0·8 (−1·0 to −0·6)
Head circumference (cm)	34·8	35·1	−0·3 (−0·4 to −0·2)
Upper abdominal circumference (cm)	33·5	34·0	−0·5 (−0·6 to −0·4)
Placental weight (g)	600	600	0 (−10 to 10)
Placental weight : birthweight ratio	18·0	17·4	0·6 (0·4–0·9)

Burnley babies is not the result of a shorter period of gestation. Nor is it explained by differences in ethnicity, social class, maternal smoking, height, age, or parity, although these account for much of the difference in head circumference.

Low ponderal index and reduced abdominal circumference at birth are followed by an increased risk of cardiovascular disease and non-insulin dependent diabetes in adult life (see chapters 3–6). Burnley has, for many years, had high death rates from cardiovascular disease, the standardised mortality ratio during 1991 being 116 compared with 90 in Salisbury. The findings in table 11.2 suggest that these high death rates will persist into the next generation. This would be consistent with Osmond's[32] long term forecasts of national and regional trends in cardiovascular mortality in England and Wales. These forecasts, based on analysis of recent trends, suggest that there will be a large fall in deaths from coronary heart disease but worsening in the differential between the north and south of the country.

Figure 11.9 shows that the lower mean ponderal index in Burnley reflects a different distribution of the measurements throughout the population and is not simply the result of an excess of very small, thin babies. The same conclusion applies to abdominal circumference.[31] The greater thinness of Burnley babies therefore results from influences which impair fetal growth throughout its whole range. The nature of these influences is largely unknown but they are presumably linked to maternal nutrition (see chapter 9).

Mothers in Salisbury, whose haemoglobin concentrations fell below 10·0 g/dl, had children whose systolic pressures at four years of age were on average 2·9 mm Hg higher than the children of mothers with higher haemoglobin concentrations.[33] Low maternal haemoglobin is known to influence placental size and function (see chapter 9). The fetus seems to be more sensitive to maternal haemoglobin concentrations, and hence to oxygen tension, than was hitherto supposed. In a recent survey of women attending the maternity hospital in Oxford (see p. 130), Godfrey[34] found

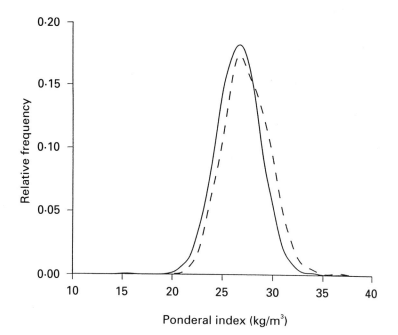

FIG 11.9—*Distribution of ponderal index (weight/length³) in newborn babies in Burnley (——) and Salisbury (– – –).*

that in 47% either the haemoglobin concentration fell below 11·0 g/dl, the WHO definition of pregnancy anaemia, or the mean red cell volume fell by more than 4 fl.[34] This suggests that iron deficiency in pregnancy remains a common condition in this country and refutes the argument that in an affluent Western country mothers are necessarily well nourished.

Government policy

The findings described in this book have profound implications for current preventive health policies. This is now recognised in Britain.[35] The Chief Medical Officer for Scotland has written:[36]

> At present we do not know whether it is more important to improve living conditions in adult life and try to persuade people to change their lifestyles, or to improve the health and nutrition of pregnant women and pre-school children. Obviously any sensible policy for improving Scotland's health must do both. But much depends on which is likely to yield greater long term benefits, and at present we do not know. We are equally ignorant about the interactions that almost certainly exist between the enduring metabolic sequelae of inadequate

nutrition early in life and unhealthy eating, drinking and exercise patterns in middle age.

The thesis of this book is that great benefit will come from improving the health and nutrition of girls and young women, and mothers during pregnancy and lactation. Developing countries do not face the same dilemma as that posed by the Chief Medical Officer. High maternal and child mortality in the developing countries necessarily focus prevention on the mother and child. The dilemma is whether greater benefit will come from improving the nutrition of girls and young women, than from improving the nutrition of young children. Hitherto interest in the nutrition and health of young women before pregnancy has been subordinated to interest in young children. This book points clearly to the need to change this emphasis.

The future

Studies of programming in fetal life and infancy are now established in the agenda for medical research. They have two goals: preventing disease in the next generation and understanding disease in the present one. The search for the causes of coronary heart disease has hitherto been guided by a "destructive" model. The causes to be identified act in adult life and accelerate destructive processes—the formation of atheroma, rise in blood pressure, loss of glucose tolerance. This book has proposed a new "developmental" model. The causes to be identified act on the baby. In adapting to them, the baby ensures its continued survival and growth at the expense of its longevity. Premature death from coronary heart disease may be viewed as the price of successful adaptations *in utero*. We need to know more about these adaptations: what they are; what induces them; how they leave a lasting mark on the body; and how this gives rise to the diseases of later life.

1 Kuh D, Davey Smith G. When is mortality risk determined? Historical insights into a current debate. *Society for the Social History of Malaise* 1993:101–23.
2 Derrick VPA. Observations on (1) Error on Age on the Population Statistics of England and Wales and (2) the changes in mortality indicated by the National Records. *Journal of the Institute of Actuaries* 1927;**58**:117–59.
3 Kermack WO, McKendrick AG, McKinlay PL. Death rates in Great Britain and Sweden. Some general regularities and their significance. *Lancet* 1934;**i**:698–703.
4 Watt GCM, Ecob R. Mortality in Glasgow and Edinburgh: a paradigm of unequality in health. *J Epidemiol Community Health* 1992;**46**:498–505.
5 Jones HB. A special consideration of the ageing process, disease and life expectancy. *Adv Biol Med Physics* 1956;**4**:281–333.
6 Watt GCM. The chief scientist report . . . Making research make a difference. *Health Bulletin* 1993;**51**:187–95.
7 McKeown T, Lowe CR. *An introduction to social medicine*. Oxford: Blackwell Scientific, 1974.
8 Barker DJP. Rise and fall of Western diseases. *Nature* 1989;**338**:371–2.

9 Office of Population Censuses and Surveys. *Registrar General's statistical review of England and Wales*. Part 1. *Tables, medical*. London: HMSO, 1880 and following years.

10 Acheson RM, Williams DRR. Epidemiology of cerebrovascular disease: some unanswered questions. In: Rose FC, ed., *Clinical neuroepidemiology*. London: Pitman Medical, 1980:88–104.

11 Barker DJP, Osmond C. Childhood respiratory infection and adult chronic bronchitis in England and Wales. *BMJ* 1986;**293**:1271–5.

12 Osmond C. Time trends in infant mortality, ischaemic heart disease and stroke in England and Wales. In: Barker DJP, ed., *Fetal and infant origins of adult disease*. London: British Medical Journal Books, 1992:119–129.

13 Lambert PM, Reid DD. Smoking, air pollution, and bronchitis in Britain. *Lancet* 1970; **i**:853–7.

14 Colley JRT, Reid DD. Urban and social origins of childhood bronchitis in England and Wales. *BMJ* 1970;**ii**:213–17.

15 Royal College of Physicians of London. *Air pollution and health*. London: Pitman, 1970.

16 Trichopoulos D. Hypothesis: does breast cancer originate in utero? *Lancet* 1990;**335**: 939–40.

17 Ekborn A, Trichopoulos D, Adami HO, Hsich CC, Lan SJ. Evidence of prenatal influences on breast cancer risk. *Lancet* 1992;**340**:1015–18.

18 Barker DJP, Osmond C, Golding J. Height and mortality in the counties of England and Wales. *Ann Hum Biol* 1990;**17**:1–6.

19 Trowell HC, Burkitt DP. *Western diseases: their emergence and prevention*. London: Arnold, 1981.

20 Phillips DIW, Barker DJP, Winter PD, Osmond C. Mortality from thyrotoxicosis in England and Wales and its association with the previous prevalence of endemic goitre. *J Epidemiol Community Health* 1983;**37**:305–9.

21 Greaves JP, Hollingsworth DF. Trends in food consumption in the United Kingdom. *World Rev Nutr Diet* 1966;**6**:34–89.

22 Barker DJP, Phillips DIW. Current incidence of thyrotoxicosis and past prevalence of goitre in 12 British towns. *Lancet* 1984;**i**:567–70.

23 Pisa Z, Uemura K. Trends of mortality from ischaemic heart disease and other cardiovascular diseases in 27 countries, 1968–1977. *World Health Stat Q* 1982;**35**: 11–47.

24 Kline J, Stein Z, Susser M. *Conception to birth—epidemiology of pre-natal development*. New York: Oxford University Press, 1976.

25 Mohan M, Shiv Prasad SR, Chellani HK, Kapani V. Intrauterine growth curves in normal Indian babies: weight, length, head circumference and ponderal index. *Indian Pediatr* 1990;**27**:43–51.

26 Centre for Health Statistics, Ministry of Public Health, People's Republic of China, 1989.

27 Ramachandran A. Epidemiology of diabetes in Indians. *International Journal of Diabetes in Developing Countries* 1993;**13**:65–7.

28 Jarrett RJ. Epidemiology and public health aspects of non-insulin dependent diabetes mellitus. *Epidemiol Rev* 1989;**11**:151–71.

29 Dowse GK, Zimmett P, Finch CF, Collins VR. Decline in incidence of epidemic glucose intolerance in Nauruans: implications for the 'thrifty genotype', *Am J Epidemiol* 1991;**133**:1093–104.

30 Marshall B, McGechie D, Rogers P, Clancy R. Pyloric campylobacter infection and gastroduodenal disease *Med J Aust* 1985;**142**:439–44.

31 Law CM, Barker DJP, Richardson WW, *et al*. Thinness at birth in a northern industrial town. *J Epidemiol Community Health* 1993;**47**:255–9.

32 Osmond C, Barker DJP. Ischaemic heart disease in England and Wales around the year 2000. *J Epidemiol Community Health* 1991;**45**:71–2.

33 Law CM, Barker DJP, Bull AR, Osmond C. Maternal and fetal influences on blood pressure. *Arch Dis Child* 1991;**66**:1291–5.

34 Godfrey KM, Redman CWG, Barker DJP, Osmond C. The effect of maternal anaemia and iron deficiency on the ratio of fetal weight to placental weight. *Br J Obstet Gynaecol* 1991;**98**:886–91.
35 Department of Health. *The health of the nation. A strategy for health in England.* London: HMSO, 1992:117.
36 Kendall R. From the Chief Medical Officer. *Health Bulletin* 1993;**51**:351–2.

Index